T0321186

CONTROVERSIES IN CARDIOVASCULAR ANESTHESIA

CONTROVERSIES IN CARDIOVASCULAR ANESTHESIA

edited by

PHILLIP N. FYMAN
ALEXANDER W. GOTTA

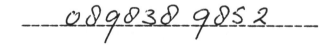

089838 9852

KLUWER ACADEMIC PUBLISHERS
Boston   Dordrecht   London

Distributors

for the United States and Canada: Kluwer Academic Publishers, 101 Philip Drive, Assinippi Park, Norwell, MA, 02061, USA

for the UK and Ireland: Kluwer Academic Publishers, Falcon House, Queen Square, Lancaster LA1 1RN, UK

for all other countries: Kluwer Academic Publishers Group, Distribution Centre, P.O. Box 322, 3300 AH Dordrecht, THE NETHERLANDS

Library of Congress Cataloging-in-Publication Data

Controversies in cardiovascular anesthesia.

Includes bibliographies and index.
1. Cardiovascular system—Surgery. 2. Anesthesia. I. Fyman,
Phillip. II. Gotta, Alexander W. [DNLM: 1. Anesthesia.
2. Cardiovascular System—surgery. WG 168 C764]
RD597.C67   1988   617'.96741   87-24774
ISBN 0-89838-985-2

We would like to acknowledge the encouragement of James Cottrell, M.D. and the support of our families, that was necessary to write this book.

Phillip N. Fyman, M.D.
Alexander W. Gotta, M.D.

CONTENTS

CONTRIBUTING AUTHORS

Enrico M. Camporesi, M.D.
  Professor of Anesthesiology
  Duke Unviersity Medical Center
  Durham, North Carolina 27710

Pierre Casthely, M.D.
  Associate Professor of Anesthesiology
  State University of New York
  Health Science Center at Brooklyn
  Brooklyn, New York

Narda Croughwell, CRNA
  Research coordinator
  Division of Cardiothoracic Anesthesia
  Duke University Medical Center
  Durham, North Carolina

John Dluzneski, M.D.
  Fellow in Cardiac Anesthesia
  State University of New York
  Health Science Center at Brooklyn
  Brooklyn, New York

Phillip N. Fyman, M.D.
Attending Anesthesiologist
Long Island Jewish Medical Center
New Hyde Park, New York 10042

Paul L. Goldiner, M.D.
Professor and Chairman
Department of Anesthesiology
Albert Einstein College of Medicine
Bronx, New York

Alexander W. Gotta, M.D.
Professor of Clinical Anesthesiology
State University of New York
Health Science Center at Brooklyn
Brooklyn, New York

Ann Govier, M.D.
Staff Anesthesiologist
Department of Cardiothoracic Anesthesia
Cleveland Clinic
Cleveland, Ohio

Jan L. Kramer, M.D.
Fellow in Cardiac Anesthesia
New York University Medical Center
New York, New York 10016

Lawrence Kushins, M.D.
Director, Cardiac Anesthesia
Long Island Jewish Medical Center
New Hyde Park, New York
    and
Clinical Assistant Professor of Anesthesiology
State University of New York
School of Medicine at Stony Brook
Stony Brook, New York

Carol L. Lake, M.D.
Associate Professor of Anesthesiology
University of Virginia School of Medicine
Charlottesville, Virginia

Martin J. London, M.D.
Assistant Professor of Anesthesiology
University of California, San Francisco
San Francisco, California

Dennis T. Mangano, Ph.D., M.D.
Professor of Anesthesiology
University of California, San Francisco
San Francisco, California

Richard E. Moon, M.D.
Assistant Professor of Anesthesiology
Duke University Medical Center
Durham, North Carolina 27710

Sarada Mylavarapu, M.D.
Fellow in Cardiac Anesthesia
Maimonides Medical Center
Brooklyn, New York 11219

Paul S. Nelson, M.D.
Fellow in Anesthesiology
University of Utah School of Medicine
Salt Lake City, Utah 84132

Yasu Oka, M.D.
Professor of Anesthesiology
Albert Einstein College of Medicine
Bronx, New York

J. G. Reves, M.D.
Professor of Anesthesiology
Director, Cardiothoracic Anesthesia
Duke University Medical Center
Durham, North Carolina

Ketan Shevde, M.D.
Director, Cardiac Anesthesia
    and
Acting Director
Department of Anesthesiology
Maimonides Medical Center
Brooklyn, New York 11219

Theodore H. Stanley, M.D.
  Professor of Anesthesiology
    and
  Research Professor of Surgery
  University of Utah School of Medicine
  Salt Lake City, Utah 84132

James B. Streisand, M.D.
  Assistant Professor of Anesthesiology
  University of Utah School of Medicine
  Salt Lake City, Utah 84132

Edward Svadjian, M.D.
  Assistant Professor of Anesthesiology
  Albert Einstein College of Medicine
  Bronx, New York

Stephen J. Thomas, M.D.
  Associate Professor of Anesthesiology
  Director of Cardiothoracic Anesthesia
  New York University Medical Center
  New York, New York 10016

David J. Wagner, M.D.
  Fellow in Cardiac Anesthesia
  New York University Medical Center
  New York, New York 10016

PREFACE

On 16 October 1846, an itinerant New England dentist named William T.G. Morton proved the anesthetic effect of diethyl ether in a public demonstration in the "ether dome" of the Bulfinch Building of the Massachusetts General Hospital in Boston. The patient, Gilbert Abbott, suffered no pain, and the surgeon, Dr. John C. Warren, was able to complete a suture ligature of a vascular tumor of the jaw without the hurry that until then was so necessary. The operation proved a failure, since the tumor recurred; but the demonstration of ether's anesthetic effect was a great success. Operative pain was conquered, and surgery could advance from a crude and unscientific practice where speed was paramount, and the major body cavities could not be entered, into the unique blend of science and art that it is now. "Gentlemen, this is no humbug," supposedly muttered Warren, perhaps the last noncontroversial assessment of anesthesiology to be made by a surgeon. The screams of resisting patients in pain were stilled, and quiet entered the operating room for the first time.

But the new science of pain relief was quickly wrapped in controversy. An argument immediately arose as to who could legitimately claim primacy for the discovery. Morton's attempt to hide the true nature of his anesthetic agent, coupled with an effort to patent the discovery, clouded his reputation and stimulated other claimants to push themselves forward. The anesthesiologists of Georgia still honor the memory of Crawford Long, while the people of Boston maintain the controversy with a monument in the Public Garden, dedicated to the discovery of ether anesthesia, yet bearing the name of no one.

While most surgeons (and all patients) readily accepted intraoperative pain relief, a few protested, claiming that pain was part of the healing process, and that to contain pain would limit healing. Fortunately, this nonsense died quickly.

Chloroform's anesthetic ability was proved only one year after the ether demonstration, and each drug's adherents trumpeted the peculiar benefits of their favorite. Chloroform, the nonflammable, but dangerous drug, with a propensity to sudden and unexplained death, became the primary agent of the physician anesthetist in Great Britain and Europe. Ether, flammable, but safer, found its greatest use in the United States.

But the infant specialty of Anesthesiology almost died in its cradle, smothered by the "religious controversy." "No!" roared the theologians of Great Britain, "you can not relieve the pain of childbirth, since the Bible demands that women shall bear their children in pain and sorrow, and it is sinful so to oppose Biblical demands." Vainly did the anesthestists protest that Adam slept while Eve was created, suggesting the divinity as the first anesthesiologist. This controversy reached a happy conclusion in 1853, when Queen Victoria received chloroform at the hands of John Snow for the delivery of Prince Leopold. Obviously, what is acceptable to the Queen and Head of the Church of England must be acceptable to all.

But controversy still exists, and arguments must be played out one against the other, conclusions drawn and repeatedly challenged. What "fact" is inviolate, what "truth" infallible? It is only in the heat of discussion that contention is tempered into truth. Controversy is necessary if we are to find our way through a maze of disjointed and seemingly unrelated facts to a modus operandi guaranteeing our patients the optimal care they deserve.

Anesthesia for cardiovascular surgery has its own range of arguments, and we have gathered opinions from a host of knowledgeable scientist-practitioners who present their viewpoints with clarity and vigor. Each presents many questions; each presents answers, contentious, controversial, debatable, but all worth pondering and considering. Come join us on a review of the controversies we consider most important. Debate with the experts, and perhaps they will help you formulate useful plans that will help you in the management of your patients.

P.N.F.

A.W.G.

CONTROVERSIES IN CARDIOVASCULAR ANESTHESIA

1. AN INHALATION ANESTHETIC TECHNIQUE IS PREFERABLE FOR PATIENTS UNDERGOING CORONARY ARTERY BYPASS GRAFTING

JAN L. KRAMER
DAVID J. WAGNER
STEPHEN J. THOMAS

What is the "best" method for anesthetizing patients for coronary artery bypass graft (CABG) surgery? Is there a "best" method? The very low morbidity and mortality reported from many centers where different anesthetics are employed [1] would suggest that there is no ideal technique. Nevertheless, it appears that the reflex response of many anesthesiologists when confronted with a patient for CABG (or for that matter any patient with "severe" heart disease) is to reach for one of the potent intravenous narcotics. To give these drugs their due, the current popularity of high-dose narcotic techniques for CABG is, no doubt, based upon their safety, the "railroad track" hemodynamics [2, 3] that often accompany their administration, and their ease of use. In many centers, volatile anesthetics have been relegated to the occasional role of treating a bit of hypertension here and there. We feel this is simplistic, inappropriate, makes little use of the beneficial properties of the vapors, and is incredibly boring. Therefore the aim of this chapter is to discuss the rationale for selecting a volatile agent as the primary anesthetic for CABG patients. We hope to encourage the intelligent use of volatile drugs by describing their safety and efficacy in patients with coronary artery disease as well as delineating potential problems or difficulties with their use.

ANESTHETIC GOALS

The anesthetic objectives for patients with coronary artery disease undergoing bypass surgery are no different from those desired for any other general anest-

1

hetic, specifically analgesia, amnesia, and suppression of untoward cardio-vascular, endocrine, and neurologic responses. The volatile anesthetics reliably meet these requirements. During the time of their administration, they provide excellent anesthesia and analgesia. Dosage can be rapidly altered to prevent or treat reflex responses to the variable levels of stimulation encountered during surgery. They are good amnestics and, when given in sufficient concentrations, prevent awareness. A potential problem in this regard is when the inspired concentration must be reduced, e.g., in the presence of poor ventricular function after cardiopulmonary bypass (CPB), it is conceivable that the patient may become aware of intraoperative events. Judicious administration of barbiturates or benzodiazepines should prevent such occurrences without interfering with the easy titratability of the volatile agent.

There are also anesthetic considerations specific to patients undergoing CABG. The presence of ischemia or the potential for developing new ischemia is obviously of prime importance. Any anesthetic drug selected should certainly not induce ischemia and, ideally, should alleviate ongoing or prevent impending episodes of new myocardial ischemia.

The deleterious effects of ischemia prior to CPB on postoperative morbidity and mortality have recently been described. Slogoff and Keats [4, 5] convincingly demonstrated that myocardial ischemia prior to CPB, whether before or after induction of anesthesia, leads to an increased incidence of postoperative myocardial infarction. In their patient population, electrocardiographic (ECG) evidence of myocardial ischemia occurred in 36.9% of all patients. Half of these episodes occurred after anesthetic induction. The incidence of postoperative myocardial infarction was nearly threefold higher (6.9% vs 2.5%) in patients demonstrating prebypass ischemia. This confirmed the earlier report by Isom et al. that emphasized the high-risk nature of the pre-CPB period and the potential for pre-CPB events causing or contributing to myocardial necrosis [6]. Therefore, prevention of prebypass ischemia in the CABG patient is extremely important. We do not have data to confirm that early treatment of isolated episodes of ischemia will also prove beneficial, but for the moment that approach seems more than reasonable.

INTRAOPERATIVE MYOCARDIAL ISCHEMIA

Merin, et al. point out that the production of ischemia by anesthetics is mediated solely by factors influencing myocardial oxygen supply and demand [7]. Anesthetics can reduce ischemia by altering the determinants of myocardial oxygen demand (wall tension, heart rate, and contractility) as well as those factors regulating coronary blood flow and its distribution (perfusion pressure, diastolic time, and coronary vascular tone).

Myocardial oxygen demand

The effects of individual volatile anesthetics on the factors determining myocardial oxygen demand (MVo_2) are presented in table 1-1. Although

Table 1-1. Cardiovascular effects of volatile anesthetics in patients with coronary artery disease

	Halothane	Enflurane	Isflurane
Hemodynamics			
Heart rate	0	0/ ↑	0/ ↑
Blood pressure	↓	↓ ↓	↓ ↓
Systemic vascular resistance	0	↓	↓ ↓
Cardiac output	↓ ↓	↓ ↓	0/ ↓
Contractility	↓ ↓	↓ ↓	↓
Myocardial energy balance			
Myocardial O_2 consumption	↓ ↓	↓ ↓	↓ ↓
Evidence of ischemia	0	0	+

there are some differences between drugs, the most important characteristic common to all is a dose-dependent depression of myocardial contractility that reduces MVO_2. The effects on wall tension are more difficult to predict. Decreased systemic arterial blood pressure due to this fall in contractility and also to vasodilation will decrease ventricular wall tension. Simultaneously, myocardial depression, if excessive, may increase wall tension by increasing ventricular end-diastolic volume. If myocardial depression is not excessive, the volatile anesthetics will generally decrease ventricular wall tension and oxygen demand. Volatile drugs have variable effects on heart rate as discussed below. In general, with the exception of isoflurane in non-beta-blocked patients, deep anesthesia is associated with a reduction in heart rate and a fall in MVO_2. As long as myocardial oxygen supply is not reduced to a greater extent than demand (i.e., hypotension-induced fall in coronary blood flow, redistribution of coronary blood flow), the potential for producing ischemia should also be reduced.

Volatile anesthetics have been shown to be efficacious in situations where ischemia is likely to develop. Bland and Lowenstein have shown that halothane can reduce signs of ischemia (ST segment change) in dogs with ligation of a branch of the left anterior descending coronary artery [8]. In addition, Roizen and colleagues have shown that hypertension and elevated filling pressures following surgical stimulation can be effectively treated with increased concentrations of a volatile anesthetic [9].

Myocardial oxygen supply

Assuming adequate levels of hemoglobin and efficient oxygenation of the blood by the lungs, myocardial oxygen supply is determined by amount and distribution of coronary blood flow. This in turn is determined by coronary perfusion pressure and coronary vascular resistance.

Coronary perfusion pressure, in the absence of luminal obstruction, is aortic pressure minus P_{ZF} (zero flow pressure). Since left ventricular subendocardial flow is essentially throttled during systole by ventricular contraction, the proximal driving pressure is aortic disastolic pressure. The driving pressure distal to a stenosis will be less than aortic diastolic pressure by a variable amount depending on severity of stenosis and flow through the stenosis. P_{ZF} refers to the end pressure in the coronary circulation—the pressure when flow falls to zero. Although the precise value P_{ZF} is somewhat controversial, it is higher than both right atrial pressure (coronary sinus pressure) and ventricular end-diastolic pressure [10]. It will be lower than this in the presence of a fixed obstruction.

Anything that *decreases* aortic diastolic pressure or *increases* P_{ZF} will reduce coronary perfusion pressure. All volatile anesthetics reduce the former. In so doing, they may induce or potentiate existing ischemia. Lowenstein and his colleagues using sonomicrometry demonstrated impaired regional wall contraction in dogs with "critical" coronary stenosis when inhaling high concentrations of halothane [11]. However, Behrenbeck et al. in an earlier study concluded that, when perfusion pressure is maintained, no differences in regional myocardial function are found [12]. Buffington [13] showed in dogs with coronary stenoses that halothane, per se, did not cause myocardial ischemia. Impaired systolic thickening during halothane anesthesia was mediated by changes in hemodynamics (specifically tachycardia or hypotension). One of the difficulties encountered in administering volatile anesthetics is determining when beneficial myocardial depression becomes deleterious hypotension-induced ischemia. This remains a dilemma because clinical monitoring devices are not yet sensitive enough to detect every episode of myocardial ischemia.

Verrier et al. have suggested that halothane may reduce P_{ZF}, increasing coronary vascular reserve [14]. Little confirmatory evidence is available, but it is possible that drugs that decrease myocardial contractility may have a small benefit for this aspect of myocardial oxygen supply.

It is apparent that myocardial depression (see below) and decreased blood pressure are inseparable attributes of volatile anesthetic agents. Is there a way for the anesthesiologist to take advantage of the decreased contractility while countering the relative hypotension and decreased blood flow to ischemic myocardia? The answer is yes, but it often requires the judicious use of vasoconstrictors to maintain the blood pressure at levels insuring adequate flow across stenotic vessels.

Myocardial depression

A major criticism of volatile anesthetics is that they are "myocardial depressants" [15]. An ischemic heart may have some degree of dysfunction and the argument is often made that further depression of contractility can only be deleterious.

This widely held opinion deserves further consideration. The ischemic heart is dysfunctional because it is ischemic; reversal of ischemia is often followed by improved function. Volatile drugs can aid in reduction of ischemia [9] by decreasing contractility and wall tension as well as by reducing heart rate through their anesthetic effects. Thus, the argument that a myocardial depressant should not be used in a dysfunctional heart becomes: a myocardial depressant can be used because the heart is ischemic and therefore dysfunctional. Anesthetics, such as the potent narcotics, that preserve myocardial function do not guarantee that the balance of myocardial oxygen supply and demand will be maintained or improved [16, 17].

Another aspect of anesthetic-induced myocardial depression (good vs bad) concerns the prime function of the heart: to provide the organs of the body with adequate amounts of oxygenated blood to meet metabolic demands. Total body oxygen consumption decreases when a patient is anesthetized, moderately hypothermic, and paralyzed as is the CABG patient. Therefore, is it necessary for the heart of this anesthetized patient to pump blood at rates that satisfied peripheral oxygen demand when awake? It would thus seem prudent to alter cardiac output in a fashion such that peripheral oxygen demand is met while minimizing myocardial oxygen demand. Volatile anesthetics are well suited to producing these effects and are thus logical choices in the patient with coronary artery disease.

Hemodynamic control

There is evidence to suggest that control of hemodynamic parameters can affect the development of perioperative ischemia and postoperative morbidity. Slogoff and Keats [4] showed that ischemia was related significantly to tachycardia. Anesthetics associated with increased rates of tachycardia and ischemia were also associated with higher rates of postoperative myocardial infarction. Rao et al. [18] showed that meticulous control of hemodynamic parameters in patients with recent myocardial infarction undergoing noncardiac surgery could significantly reduce the incidence of perioperative reinfarction. These studies suggest that control of the "numbers" can reduce the incidence of myocardial ischemia and infarction seen in patients with coronary artery disease.

It is readily apparent that volatile anesthetics can be used safely in the presence of coronary artery disease provided that meticulous attention is paid to control of heart rate (fairly slow) and coronary perfusion pressure (75% of awake values have been used in a series of studies and have been demonstrated to be adequate [17]). If these aspects of myocardial [19] oxygen supply and demand are controlled, then volatile anesthetics can be used without hesitation in coronary patients. It should be noted that control of these variables may require considerable hemodynamic manipulations by the anesthesiologist and necessitates the aggressive use of vasoactive drugs. Specific aspects of each of the volatile anesthetics in common use with respect to patients with coronary artery disease follow.

HALOTHANE

Moffitt et al. [20] studied six patients with preserved left ventricular function undergoing CABG with halothane as the major anesthetic. The dose of halothane was titrated to keep the systolic pressure slightly below awake values.

Mean arterial blood pressure decreased 17%. No change from awake values occurred in heart rate, systemic vascular resistance, or cardiac index. Coronary sinus flow (measured by thermodilution) was unchanged, but myocardial oxygen consumption decreased by 34%. No ischemia was noted and myocardial lactate extraction (a measure of aerobic metabolism) continued.

Reiz et al. [21] studied ten patients with stable ischemic heart disease and moderate heart failure. Halothane was administered at a 1% end-tidal level to patients prior to undergoing vascular surgery. Mean arterial pressure (−42%), systemic vascular resistance (−39%), and cardiac index (−20%) all decreased. Coronary sinus blood flow (thermodilution method) decreased in parallel to the perfusion pressure. Myocardial oxygen consumption decreased by 60% and there was continued myocardial lactate extraction, indicating absence of anaerobic metabolism and ischemia.

Halothane appears to be an acceptable agent for CABG patients for several reasons. It is a good myocardial depressant and is generally felt to cause less direct vasodilation than the other agents. Thus, coronary perfusion pressure may be more easily maintained. Tachycardia is generally not a problem during halothane anesthesia. For these reasons, halothane can provide conditions promoting a favorable myocardial supply–demand balance, thus preventing or alleviating ischemia.

ENFLURANE

Enflurane is similar to halothane in its ability to lower determinants of myocardial oxygen demand. The mechanism of decreased oxygen demand, however, differs slightly between the two agents. Delaney et al. [22] demonstrated that, in patients with good ventricular function and coronary artery disease, halothane caused more myocardial depression and enflurane caused more decrease in afterload. Another study, however, showed that enflurane, like halothane, decreased myocardial oxygen demand by direct myocardial depression. In ten patients, most of whom were beta-blocked, with good ventricular function undergoing coronary artery bypass surgery, Moffit et al. [23] found that enflurane reduced mean arterial pressure by ~35% and this was due solely to a decrease in cardiac index approximately (−30%) as systemic vascular resistance did not change. Coronary sinus blood flow decreased by about 30% while myocardial oxygen consumption decreased by about 50%, indicating improvement in the myocardial oxygen supply–demand balance. No change was noted in myocardial lactate extraction and no clinical signs of ischemia occurred.

Rydvall et al. [24] found that enflurane had similar hemodynamic effects to those found by Delaney et al. [22]. Enflurane decreased mean arterial pressure (−50%) predominately through vasodilation (systemic vascular resistance −41% vs cardiac index −27%). Myocardial oxygen consumption decreased 40% while coronary sinus flood flow decreased 29%. Despite this apparent improvement in myocardial oxygen balance, four of 11 patients showed clinical signs of ischemia and demonstrated decreased lactate extraction or lactate production. This study was unable to differentiate between redistribution of coronary blood flow caused by enflurane-induced coronary vasodilation and hypotension leading to reduced flow across a coronary artery stenosis as a cause of the ischemia. This latter study by Rydvall et al. [24] emphasizes the necessity for hemodynamic control during anesthesia with volatile agents. Enflurane appears to be a satisfactory agent and can be safely used with the proviso that tight hemodynamic control is maintained.

ISOFLURANE

Isoflurane is a myocardial depressant, though less than either enflurane or halothane. It produces dose-dependent decreases in left ventricular function and hence oxygen consumption [25]. Tachycardia in non-beta-blocked patients is dose dependent and is likely due to preserved baroreceptor function in the face of peripheral vasodilation, one of the major effects of isoflurane. It is now fairly well established that isoflurane is a potent dilator of small resistance vessels in the coronary circulation, more so than enflurane or halothane [26–28]. It is this property and the presumed site of action of isoflurane that may lead to a coronary "steal" and the production of myocardial ischemia.

Reiz et al. [27] investigated the hemodynamic and myocardial metabolic effects of an isoflurane–nitrous oxide mixture in 21 patients with stable angina. Mean arterial pressure decreased ~30%, heart rate increased slightly, and cardiac index decreased slightly. Coronary perfusion pressure (defined as diastolic blood pressure minus pulmonary wedge pressure) decreased by 35%, as did myocardial oxygen consumption. Coronary sinus blood flow was unchanged, indicating a decrease in coronary vascular resistance. Ten of the 21 patients had ECG evidence of new ischemia. In these patients, myocardial lactate extraction decreased by 52% compared to the patients who had no clinical evidence of ischemia. In the last ten patients in this series, coronary perfusion pressure was returned to awake values by a phenylephrine infusion. Five of these patients had become ischemic. In two of these patients, the ischemia persisted despite return of hemodynamic parameters to preanesthetic levels. In these patients, the decrease in coronary vascular resistance in combination with clinical and metabolic evidence of ischemia points indirectly toward the production of a coronary "steal." Moffit et al. [28] studied a similar group of patients undergoing coronary bypass surgery and found similar hemodynamic changes. Three of ten patients demonstrated clinical and metabolic evidence of ischemia (ECG changes, decreased myocardial lactate extraction). Larsen et al. [29] demonstrated similar hemodynamics and a similar 30% incidence of ischemia in coronary patients anesthetized with isoflurane.

Isoflurane in lower doses has not been associated with a high incidence of ischemia. Tarnow et al. [30] described improved tolerance to pacing-induced myocardial ischemia during 0.5% isoflurane–50% nitrous oxide in oxygen.

Smith et al. [31] compared two groups of patients with impaired ventricular function undergoing coronary bypass surgery. One group received high-dose fentanyl and the other a lower dose of fentanyl plus 0.5%–1.0% isoflurane. No difference in incidence of myocardial ischemia was seen. Recent studies have shown no or minimal ischemia at low (i.e., less than 1 MAC) concentrations of isoflurane (S. Reiz, personal communication).

Two recent animal studies demonstrate the effect of isoflurane on the distribution of coronary blood flow. Buffington et al. [32] measured regional blood flow in a dog with a chronic stenosis of the left anterior descending artery. They found that isoflurane decreased blood flow to the region supplied by the chronically stenosed artery, while at the same time increasing flow through nonstenosed arteries. In addition, isoflurane induced an alteration in transmural distribution of flow such that the subepicardium was perfused at the expense of the subendocardium in both ischemic and normal areas. Neither halothane nor nitrous oxide produced similar changes. Sill et al. [33] measured coronary artery dimensions angiographically and coronary blood flow and myocardial oxygen consumption over a range of isoflurane concentrations (0.75%–2.25%). They were unable to find any difference in epicardial artery dimensions, yet coronary blood flow increased in a dose-dependent manner, indicating the site of dilation to be at the level of the arteriole. Becker [34] points out that compounds that dilate coronary arterioles are known to be capable of producing ischemia through a coronary "steal" mechanism.

It is apparent that isoflurane as the sole anesthetic agent can cause myocardial ischemia in patients with coronary artery disease even in the presence of a normal hemodynamic state. That this ischemia is the result of a maldistribution of coronary blood flow is only slightly less apparent. Other aspects of isoflurane may make this agent less efficacious for patients with coronary artery disease. Tendencies toward tachycardia and decreased coronary perfusion pressure may require the use of vasoactive drugs. However, when used in low doses (0.5% end-tidal concentration) and as part of a mixed technique and under carefully monitored situations, isoflurane does not appear to cause ischemia.

SURGICAL REQUIREMENTS

Specific aspects of CABG deserve consideration during the design of an anesthetic plan. This operation has distinct periods, each of which imposes particular demands and constraints upon the anesthesiologist.

During the prebypass period, there are brief, but intense, periods of autonomic stimulation (intubation, sternotomy, aortic mobilization, and cannulation). The volatile anesthetics can easily be titrated in anticipation of these events in order to prevent untoward hemodynamic responses. These agents are capable of suppressing autonomic responses far better than are narcotics, which often allow hypertension and tachycardia to occur. Unlike the intravenous narcotics, once the brief period of stimulation is passed, the volatile drug can easily be eliminated to better suit the ongoing level of stimulation.

During CPB, the patient's body temperature is usually lowered, thus decreasing anesthetic requirements. A minimum, but steady, level of anesthetic must be maintained to prevent awareness. This requires the presence of a vaporizer in the oxygenator circuit. The volatile agent may also be used to attenuate the well-described autonomic hyperactivity induced by CPB, as well as to enable easy control of systemic vascular resistance and blood pressure.

The post-CPB period is initially one of unpredictability and variability of myocardial function. It is during this time that volatile anesthetics may cause problems by virtue of their myocardial depressant actions. After separation from CPB, careful evaluation of cardiac performance is mandatory. Volatile drugs should only be used when contractility is good and mild depression of function will be tolerated. If contractility is marginal, then volatile agents should not be used; alternative amnesics and anesthetics should then be selected.

In the early postoperative period, the speed with which volatile anesthetics are eliminated allows the patient to awaken and breathe earlier [35] than after a narcotic anesthetic. Spontaneous ventilation may help improve the patient's hemodynamics primarily by augmenting venous return to the heart. The rapid elimination of volatile anesthetics assures that the patient will require analgesics in the early postoperative period to prevent pain-induced tachycardia and hypertension. While the lack of postoperative pain relief provided by volatile agents is clearly a negative aspect, the ability to titrate analgesics to patient needs in the intensive care unit clearly adds a degree of flexibility unavailable with narcotic anesthetics.

CONCLUSION

The choice of anesthetic for coronary artery bypass surgery can significantly affect the morbidity and outcome of the procedure. Adequate control of factors determining myocardial oxygen supply and demand minimizes the risk of ischemia developing prior to CPB and can reduce the incidence of postoperative infarction. The volatile anesthetics, with the likely exception of isoflurane, can influence the myocardial oxygen supply–demand balance in favor of preventing ischemia. They do this by decreasing myocardial contractility, afterload and, most cases, heart rate. They are potentially harmful in that decreased coronary perfusion pressure almost uniformly occurs. One very important aspect of these drugs is that meticulous attention to hemodynamic control is required. In order to maintain coronary perfusion, it is often necessary to use vasoactive drugs and drugs that alter heart rate. This is compared to the narcotic anesthetic in which blood pressure and heart rate rarely change. So why use volatile agents at all? These agents provide good suppression of sympathetic responses, they are easily titratable, and they can allow early awakening and extubation. They are also myocardial depressants that, per se, are usually beneficial as long as the accompanying decrease in coronary perfusion pressure is not allowed to reach intolerable limits. Myocardial depression decreases oxygen demand, which, in an ischemic heart, can only be good (within limits, of course).

Isoflurane presents the anesthesiologist with a dilemma. Ostensibly the agent should be good for an ischemic heart. It is a mild myocardial depressant and a potent vasodilator. Over the past four years, however, a large body of evidence has accumulated strongly suggesting that isoflurane can cause ischemia by redistributing coronary blood flow. Isoflurane should be avoided whenever coronary blood flow is largely via collateral vessels. It should be turned off whenever tachycardia or significant hypotension occurs during its use. It is likely that at low concentrations the drug is probably safe. More vehement critics would suggest that, as long as the potential for coronary redistribution exists, isoflurane should never be used in patients with coronary disease. The ultimate decision in this controversy must await the results of outcome studies that are currently in progress. Studies elucidating the mechanisms of isoflurane-induced ischemia are beginning to be published. Further work is required to delineate these mechanisms.

Where does this leave the anesthesiologist who wants to anesthetize the patient safely, provide good hemodynamic control, and hasten recovery? To reiterate our opening question—is there a "best" method. The answer is: probably not. We feel that volatile anesthetics have a major role in the anesthesia for CABG patients. Their attributes that lead to reduction in ischemia make them almost indispensible for this type of surgery. They are not the whole answer, however. We feel that, in combination with small amounts of the potent narcotics, the volatile anesthetics can be used with great success and safety.

REFERENCES

1. Miller DC, Stinson EB, Oyer PE, et al.: Discriminant analysis of the changing risks of coronary artery operations: 1971–1979. J Thorac Cardiovasc Surg 85:197, 1983.
2. Delange S, Boscoe MJ, Stanley TH: Comparison of sufentanil–O_2 and fentanyl–O_2 for coronary artery surgery. Anesthesiology 56:112, 1982.
3. Stanley TH, Webster LR: Anesthetic requirements and cardiovascular effects of fentanyl–O_2 and fentanyl–diazepam–O_2 anesthesia in man. Anesth Analg 57:411, 1978.
4. Slogoff S, Keats AS: Does perioperative myocardial ischemia lead to postoperative myocardial infarction? Anesthesiology 62:107, 1985.
5. Slogoff S, Keats AS: Further observations on perioperative myocardial ischemia. Anesthesiology 65:539, 1986.
6. Isom OW, Spencer FC, Feigenbaum H, Cunningham Jn Jr, Roe C: Prebypass myocardial damage in patients undergoing coronary revascularization: an unrecognized vulnerable period. Circulation [Suppl] 52:II–119, 1975.
7. Merin, RG, Lowenstein E, Gelman S: Is anesthesia beneficial for the ischemic heart? III. Anesthesiology 64:137, 1986.
8. Bland JHL, Lowenstein E: Halothane induced decrease in experimental myocardial ischemia in the non-failing canine heart. Anesthesiology 45:287, 1976.
9. Roizen MF, Hamilton WK, Yung JS: Treatment of stress-induced increases in pulmonary capillary wedge pressure using volatile anesthetics. Anesthesiology 55:446–450, 1981.
10. Dole WP, Alexander GM, Campbell AB, Hixson EL, Bishop VS: Interpretation and physiological significance of diastolic coronary artery pressure–flow relationships in the canine coronary bed. Cir Res 55:215–226, 1984.

11. Lowenstein E, Foex P, Francis CM, Davies WL, Yusuf S, Ryder WA: Regional ischemic ventricular dysfunction in myocardium supplied by a narrowed coronary artery with increasing halothane concentration in the dog. Anesthesiology 55:349, 1981.
12. Behrenbeck T, Nugent M, Quasha A, Hoffman E, Ritman E, Tinker J: Halothane and ischemic regional myocardial wall dynamics. Anesthesiology 53:5140, 1980.
13. Buffington CW: Impaired systolic thickening associated with halothane in the presence of a coronary stenosis is mediated by changes in hemodynamics. Anesthesiology 64:632, 1986.
14. Verrier ED, Edelist G, Consigny PM, Robinson S, Hotfman JIE: Greater coronary vascular reserve in dogs anestheticed with halothane. Anesthesiology 53:445–459, 1980.
15. Merin RG: Are the myocardial functional and metabolic effects of isoflurane really different from those of halothane and enflurane? Anesthesiology 55:398, 1981.
16. Sonntag H, Larsen R, Hilfiker O, Kettler D, Brockschnieder B: Myocardial blood flow and oxygen consumption during high dose fentanyl anesthesia in patients with coronary artery disease. Anesthesiology 56:417, 1982.
17. Moffit EA, Scovil JE, Barker RA: Myocardial metabolism and hemodynamic response during high dose fentanyl anesthesia for coronary patients. Can Anaesth Soc J 31:611, 1984.
18. Rao TLK, Jacobs KH, El-Etr AA: Reinfarction following anesthesia in patients with myocardial infarction. Anesthesiology 58:499–505, 1983.
19. Moffitt EA, Sethna DH: The coronary circulation and myocardial oxygenation in coronary artery disease: effects of anesthesia. Anesth Analg 65:395, 1986.
20. Moffitt EA, Sethna DH, Bussell JA, Raymond M, Matloff JM, Gray RJ: Myocardial metabolism and hemodynamic responses to halothane or morphine anesthesia for coronary artery surgery. Anesth Analg 61:979, 1982.
21. Reiz S, Balfors E, Gustavsson B, Haggmark S, Nath S, Rydvall A, Truedsson H: Effects of halothane on coronary hemodynamics and ischemic heart disease and heart failure. Acta Anaesthesiol Scand 26:133, 1982.
22. Delaney TJ, Kistner JR, Lake CL, Miller ED: Myocardial function during halothane and enflurane anesthesia in patients with coronary artery disease. Anesth Analg 59:240, 1980.
23. Moffit EA, Imrie DD, Scovil JE, Glenn JJ, Couisins CL, DelCampo C, Sullivan JA, Kinley CE: Myocardial metabolism and haemodynamic responses with enflurane anesthesia for coronary artery surgery. Can Anaesth Soc J 31:604, 1984.
24. Rydvall A, Haggmark S, Nyhman H, Reiz S: Effects of enflurane on coronary hemodynamics in patients with ischemic heart disease. Acta Anaesthesiol Scand 28:690, 1984.
25. Eger II EI: Isoflurane: a review. Anesthesiology 55:559, 1981.
26. Gelman S, Fowler KC, Smith LR: Regional blood flow during isoflurane and halothane anesthesia. Acta Anaesthesiol Scand 63:557, 1984.
27. Reiz S, Balfors E, Sorensen MB, Ariola S, Friedman A, Truedsson H: Isoflurane: a powerful coronary vasodilator in patients with coronary artery disease. Anesthesiology 59:91, 1983.
28. Moffit EA, Barker RA, Glenn JJ, Imrie DD, Delcampo C, Landymore RW, Kinley CE, Murphy DP: Myocardial metabolism and hemodynamic responses with isoflurane anesthesia for coronary arterial surgery. Anesth Analg 65:53, 1986.
29. Larsen R, Hilfiker O, Merkel G, Sonntag H, Drobnik L: Myocardial oxygen balance during enflurane and isoflurane anesthesia for coronary artery surgery [abstr]. Anesthesiology 61:A4, 1984.
30. Tarnow J, Markschies-Horning A, Schulte-Sasse V: Isoflurane increases the tolerance to pacing induced myocardial ischemia. Anesthesiology 64:147, 1986.
31. Smith JS, Cahalan MK, Benefiel DJ, Lurz FW, Lampe GH, Byrd BJ, Schiller NB, Yee ES, Turley K, Ullyot DJ, Hamilton WR: Fentanyl versus fentanyl–isoflurane in patients with impaired left ventricular function. [abstr]. Anesthesiology 63:A3, 1985.
32. Buffington CW, Romson JL, Leven A, Duttlinger NC, Huang AW: Isoflurane induces coronary steal in a canine model of chronic coronary occlusion. Anesthesiology 66:280, 1987.
33. Sill JC, Bove AA, Nugent M, Blaise GA, Dewey JD, Griban C: Effects of isoflurane on coronary arteries and coronary arterioles in the dog. Anesthesiology 66:262, 1987.
34. Becker LC: Is isoflurane dangerous for the patient with coronary artery disease? Anesthesiology 66:259, 1987.
35. Lichtenthal PR, Wade LD, Niemyski R, Shapiro BA: Respiratory management after cardiac surgery with inhalation anesthesia. Crit Care Med 11:603, 1983.

2. AN INTRAVENEOUS TECHNIQUE IS PREFERABLE FOR PATIENTS UNDERGOING CORONARY ARTERY BYPASS GRAFTING

JAMES B. STREISAND
THEODORE H. STANLEY
PAUL S. NELSON

The rapid growth of cardiac surgery during the last two decades has required the anesthesiologist to provide anesthetic regimens that impart safety and favorable outcome to patients with cardiovascular disease. This has stimulated research and clinical testing of a variety of anesthetic drugs and techniques to determine which, if any, is best for patients with coronary artery disease (CAD) undergoing coronary artery bypass grafting (CABG). Two schools of thought have emerged. One favors potent inhalational agents as the primary anesthetic for CABG while the other considers intravenous agents to be superior. Thus, the question arises: is there data that document advantages of intravenous or inhalational agents as the primary anesthetic for CABG patients?

Some investigators have attempted to answer this question with prospective, controlled, clinical studies. While differences in some physiologic variables have been reported, morbidity with cardiovascular surgery has not been correlated with specific anesthetic technique(s). [1] A variety of studies have compared hemodynamic and myocardial [2–11], endocrine [4, 7, 11], and renal [12] function in patients undergoing cardiac surgery with narcotic- and inhalational-based anesthesia. While many reports show physiologic function more satisfactory with narcotic-based techniques [2–4, 7], no improvement in patient outcome has been convincingly associated with either technique. This may be due in part to the relatively low morbidity and mortality rates associated with CABG procedures regardless of anesthetic technique. When small differences in outcome are associated with a particular technique, very large numbers of patients are required for a study to demonstrate statistical significance [1].

Although it has not yet been possible to prove rigorously the advantage of one anesthetic technique over another, recent studies have documented that anesthesiologists and anesthetic techniques do affect patient morbidity [13, 14]. Indeed, Slogoff and Keats [13] showed an 11-fold difference in postoperative myocardial infarction rates among CABG patients managed by nine different anesthesiologists (table 2-1). This report found strong associations between intraoperative tachycardia and myocardial ischemia and perioperative morbidity (myocardial infarction). These data confirm the fact that hemodynamic stability is of paramount importance in anesthetic cardiovascular management. The results also provide evidence that much can be gained by examining the effects of anesthetic technique on pathophysiologic variables pertinent to outcome following coronary artery bypass surgery.

Narcotic-based intravenous anesthetic regimens are frequently utilized today in the care of operative patients with significant cardiovascular dysfunction. While a variety of anesthetic techniques—inhalation, intravenous, or combinations of the two—are successfully used in patients with poor cardiac performance, intravenous narcotic agents provide several distinct advantages. First of all, narcotic analgesics provide remarkable hemodynamic stability, cause little cardiac depression, and significantly attenuate hormonal stress responses to surgery. Central nervous system circulatory autoregulation is also maintained with narcotic anesthesia and, if required, reversal agents (nalbuphine, naloxone) are available [15–17].

Table 2-1. Role of anesthesiology in perioperative ischemia and perioperative myocardial infarction (PMI)

| Anesthesiologist | No. of patients | Incidence (%) during anesthesia | | | |
		Ischemia	PMI	Tachycardia	Hypertension
1	139	29	2.9	19	9
2	131	22	4.6	21	5
3	104	26	3.8	23	11
4	118	38*	5.1	27	14
5	138	18	5.1	20	8
6	129	22	3.1	23	4
7	64	45*	12.5*	48*	17*
8	105	32	1.9	28	16*
9	95	26	1.1	24	5
Total	1023	27.6	4.1	24.3	9.4
Multiple chi-square		<0.0005	<0.05	<0.005	<0.01

*Significantly greater than group mean ($p < 0.05$).
From Slogoff and Keats [13].

This chapter examines the theoretical and practical considerations of employing narcotic analgesics (opioids) and other intravenous compounds as primary anesthetics for patients undergoing CABG surgery. Their advantages and disadvantages are compared to those of inhalational anesthetic techniques.

PREOPERATIVE CONSIDERATIONS

Planning the anesthetic technique for CABG patients requires a thorough understanding of the patient's preoperative pathophysiologic state as well as the surgical procedure. Each patient presents new and unique problems to the anesthesiologist. Preoperative factors that may influence the anesthetic plan include the patient's myocardial function and concurrent medical therapy.

Myocardial function

One of the most important preoperative factors in planning an anesthetic technique is myocardial function. Patients awaiting coronary artery surgery who have a history of congestive heart failure or an ejection fraction of less than 0.5 have an increased incidence of operative mortality [18]. Perioperative decreases in myocardial performance leading to decreases in cardiac output may endanger perfusion of vital organs such as the heart, brain, and kidney during operation and cause postoperative dysfunction. Therefore, it is necessary to choose an anesthetic technique that minimizes perturbations of these vital organ systems without increasing myocardial metabolic requirements or reducing coronary blood flow.

Patients with coronary artery disease undergoing coronary artery bypass procedures are often classified according to their level of myocardial function [19] (table 2-2). In patients with normal ventricular function, myocardial ischemia more frequently results secondary to hypertension, tachycardia, arrhythmias, and/or coronary artery spasm. Thus, anesthetic techniques that inhibit or minimize sympathetic responses to stimulation are desirable. How-

Table 2-2. Two groups of patients with atherosclerotic cardiovascular disease

Group 1: coronary artery disease but good ventricular function
  Angina pectoris is primary symptom; may have features of coronary artery spasm
  Hypertension frequently associated
  Cardiac index normal; ejection fraction >0.55
  Left ventricular end-diastolic pressure <12 mmHg
  No ventricular wall motion abnormalities

Group 2: coronary artery disease and poor ventricular function
  Symptoms of congestive heart failure are prominent complaint
  Little or no cardiac reserve
  Previous myocardial infarction(s)
  Cardiac index <2 L/min/m²; ejection fraction <0.4
  Left ventricular end-diastolic pressure >18 mmHg
  Hypokinetic or dyskinetic (aneurysmal) segments of ventricle

From Clark and Stanley [19].

ever, in patients with CAD and associated hypodynamic ventricular function, congestive heart failure may be the principal predisposing factor in myocardial ischemia. This latter group of patients will benefit from an anesthetic technique that preserves myocardial contractility and left ventricular (LV) function.

The new synthetic opioids fentanyl and sufentanil are effective in meeting the requirements of both groups of patients. Intraoperative utilization of these intravenous agents provides a deep level of anesthesia with effective blunting of surgical stimuli [20–23]. Some authors advocate the use of inhalational agents in the patient population with good LV function in order to reduce myocardial oxygen requirements [24]. However, cardiovascular depression and vascular dilation caused by these agents often produce a transient fall in mean arterial blood pressure and a subsequent reduction in coronary perfusion pressure [25]. These changes may lead to significant decreases in blood flow to areas of the heart distal to the stenotic coronary artery lesion(s).

Isoflurane has been shown to be a potent coronary vasodilator. Reiz and others [26, 27] have shown that a "coronary steal" may potentially develop with the use of these agents in the presence of coronary artery stenosis. This phenomenon results in a significant reduction in blood flow in the areas distal to the stenosis with redistribution to those areas with normal coronary vasculature. Thus, the use of inhalational agents to decrease myocardial oxygen demand may result in ischemia in those areas of the heart at greatest risk for low blood flow.

Patients with poor ventricular function are at risk of LV failure and pulmonary congestion when inhalational agents are used as the primary anesthetic for CABG surgery. The resulting depression of myocardial function and loss of sympathetic tone associated with these agents may lead to hemodynamic instability and inadequate perfusion of vital organs. These patients obviously require an anesthetic technique that maintains LV function and tissue perfusion. Intravenous opioid anesthesia with fentanyl or sufentanil more readily achieves this desired goal [21, 23, 28]. With careful titration of these agents, adequate anesthetic depth may be obtained without cardiac decompensation. Although both inhalation and intravenous techniques continue to be used successfully in patients with poor LV function, the hemodynamic stability provided by the new synthetic opioids has made the use of inhalation agents less common [29].

Concurrent drug therapy

Patients awaiting coronary artery bypass surgery are often taking a wide variety of medications. Current medical management of coronary artery disease often includes beta-blockers and calcium channel blockers. Additional antihypertensive therapy is also frequently required in this patient population. As current anesthetic practice involves the continuation of medical therapy up until the morning of surgery, possible interactions with anesthetic agents must be evaluated prior to selecting an anesthetic technique.

Beta-blockers

Chronic treatment with propranolol has been shown to decrease narcotic requirements during CABG and provide a smoother intraoperative course in those patients with good LV function [30]. Studies have also demonstrated significant bradycardia following opioid induction in patients with beta-blockade [20]. In patients with marginal ventricular function who are dependent upon heart rate to maintain cardiac output, myocardial ischemia may result if adequate therapy to restore baseline heart rate is not rapidly initiated. In this patient population, an anticholinergic agent can be given as a premedication or upon arrival in the operating room to attenuate the bradycardia sometimes seen with narcotic inductions [30, 31].

Calcium channel blockers

Patients with CAD who present for CABG are not uncommonly taking calcium-channel-blocking agents on a chronic basis. Conflicting reports regarding the use of narcotic anesthesia in patients on chronic calcium-channel-blocker regimens have appeared in the medical literature. An initial report associating high-dose fentanyl anesthesia with severe hypotension in patients using nifedipine resulted in recommendations for the discontinuation of nifedipine 36 h prior to CABG (with fentanyl anesthesia) [32]. This drug interaction may result from fentanyl's interference with the compensatory sympathetic reflexes needed to counteract the vasodilation and myocardial depression caused by nifedipine [33]. In contrast, Roach et al. found no evidence of hemodynamic instability during fentanyl anesthesia in patients on chronic nifedipine therapy [34]. Casson et al. also observed no increased incidence of hypotension in patients continuing their nifedipine regimen up to the day of (CABG) surgery [35]. Likewise, continuation of diltiazem therapy has not been associated with significant hemodynamic changes during intravenous narcotic anesthesia for CABG surgery [36]. Early withdrawal of calcium channel blockers may cause myocardial ischemia, coronary artery spasm, and rebound hypertension [37]. In addition, patients whose nifedipine therapy is withdrawn preoperatively often have an increased requirement for vasodilators to treat hypertension after bypass and in the postoperative period [35]. Thus, the risks associated with acute withdrawal of calcium channel blockers appear to be significant whereas hemodynamic instability is rare when patients taking calcium channel blockers are given high doses of opioids. Therefore, the data suggest that continuation of calcium-channel-blocker therapy during the preoperative period is advisable whenever intravenous narcotic anesthetic techniques are utilized for CABG procedures.

Since inhalation anesthetics and calcium channel blockers both depress myocardial contractility and smooth muscle reactivity by altering calcium flux across cell membranes, the potential for drug interaction is significant [38, 39]. Animal studies have demonstrated enhanced hemodynamic depression when a volatile anesthetic is administered in the presence of verapamil or diltiazem

[40–45]. In addition, this combination of agents in dogs has been associated with prolongation of atrioventricular conduction, second-degree heart block, junctional rhythm, and sinoatrial node arrest [44, 45]. Studies using the isolated rat heart preparation have shown nifedipine and halothane to be synergistic in their depression of myocardial contractility [46]. Data from these studies imply the possibility of potentially dangerous interactions between inhalation anesthetic agents and the calcium channel blockers, and suggest that caution be taken when they are used in combination in patients with cardiovascular dysfunction [47].

Antihypertensive agents

It is well known that antihypertensive agents that act within the central nervous system by depressing sympathetic outflow (alpha-methyldopa, reserpine, and clonidine, for example) decrease minimum alveolar concentration (MAC) requirements for inhalation agents [48–50]. A recent report demonstrated that a single dose of clonidine given preoperatively reduces fentanyl requirements for CABG surgery by up to 45% and provides a smoother intraoperative course [51]. Similarly, chronic propranolol therapy significantly reduces fentanyl, sufentanil, and other narcotic requirements [30]. Changes in intravenous narcotic requirements in patients taking potent antihypertensive drugs must be anticipated when planning the anesthetic management of cardiac surgery patients. Careful titration of narcotics to produce desired clinical effects minimizes potential untoward effects resulting from their interaction with other drugs and avoids overdosage and prolonged anesthesia.

CABG SURGERY

Induction and maintenance of anesthesia

Patients with significant, uncorrected coronary artery disease who undergo CABG surgery are at high risk for myocardial ischemia during and following induction of anesthesia until cardiopulmonary bypass. The challenge of maintaining optimal myocardial oxygen balance is complicated by the "peaks and valleys" in somatic and sympathetic nervous system stimulation associated with endotracheal intubation, skin incision, sternal split and spread, manipulation of the aortic arch, and aortic cannulation. An adequate anesthetic technique must control sympathethic reflex activity. In addition, the anesthetic must preserve vascular and myocardial function and vital organ perfusion during the time intervals between stimulation. Although a variety of agents and techniques have been used to meet these demands, narcotics have proven to be particularly valuable.

Morphine was the first narcotic employed as an anesthetic agent for cardiac surgery. Lowenstein et al., in 1969, used morphine in intravenous doses ranging from 0.6 to 3.0 mg/kg to anesthetize severely ill patients undergoing cardiac valvular replacement [52]. Due to morphine's lack of cardiovascular depression, it soon became popular for use in a variety of cardiac surgical procedures, including CABG. With increasing usage, however, many clinicians began experiencing serious problems with morphine anesthesia. Dalton [53], Stoelting and Gibbs [54], and Kistner et al. [3] were among several who reported "breakthrough" hypertension and tachycardia with resultant myocardial ischemia at numerous times during CABG. A high incidence of intraoperative awareness, significant increases in plasma histamine levels, and prolonged postoperative respiratory depression also proved to be problematic. The undesired effects associated with morphine anesthesia in patients with cardiovascular disease prompted investigation into the development of the new synthetic narcotics for use in cardiac surgery.

In 1978, Stanley and Webster first reported their experience with fentanyl and 100% oxygen as a complete anesthetic for cardiac surgery. Patients with severe mitral valve dysfunction received 8–15 µg/kg fentanyl for induction and loss of consciousness, with an average of 74 µg/kg required for the entire operation [31]. In a subsequent study, 71 µg/kg fentanyl was used for coronary artery surgery [55]. These initial studies demonstrated fentanyl's ability to provide stable cardiovascular hemodynamics when used as the primary anesthetic agent for cardiac surgery. Since many of the problems associated with the use of morphine have not been reported following fentanyl administration, its use as an anesthetic for cardiac surgery has become widespread.

Fentanyl dosage requirements for induction of anesthesia in patients undergoing CABG as well as the optimal rate of administration have been and remain controversial. Fentanyl (unlike morphine) may be administered rapidly, without histamine release, venodilation, and resultant hypotension [20]. Therefore, may clinicians infuse fentanyl as a single, large, precalculated bolus of 500–100 µg/kg for induction and maintenance of anesthesia. While this technique has proven somewhat satisfactory, careful titration of anesthetic dose to desired clinical effect (loss of consciousness, blunted sympathetic reflexes, stable heart rate, and blood pressure) is optimal. As opioids exhibit a significant degree of dose-response variability, administration methods that titrate drug dose to clinical effect are preferred.

Stanley and de Lange evaluated the effect of tobacco, alcohol, and caffeine consumption on fentanyl requirements during CABG. Patients with a history of using these agents required significantly more fentanyl than did the control group, and had a higher incidence of side effects (rigidity 80% vs 10% and hypertension 40% vs 0%) [56]. In another study, patients who underwent CABG in Leiden, the Netherlands, were reported to require greater amounts of fentanyl for induction and maintenance of anesthesia than did a similar group of patients in Salt Lake City, Utah [57]. As indicated by these observations, variability in patient response to any given narcotic dose must be anticipated, and smoking, and alcohol, and/or caffeine consumption should be viewed as additional factors that affect fentanyl requirements for CABG surgery.

A variety of fentanyl-dosing regimens have been used for induction and maintenance of anesthesia during cardiac surgery. The anesthetic dose of fentanyl is often determined empirically and administered as a single bolus at the time of induction. Fentanyl should be carefully titrated at a rate of 200–400 µg/min until loss of consciousness occurs (indicated by lack of response to verbal commands), and then administered slowly (with a muscle relaxant) to deepen anesthesia and eliminate sympathetic response to laryngoscopy and tracheal intubation. Small, intermittent boluses of fentanyl (200–400 µg) are then administered as required for control of hemodynamic response to surgical stimulation. When fentanyl is slowly titrated in this manner, severe hypotension and bradycardia are rare [21, 31, 55, 56, 58, 59].

Yet another regimen uses a continuous opioid infusion following induction in an attempt to maintain steady plasma drug levels [60–63]. An infusion has theoretical and practical advantages over single or intermittent bolus techniques. The ability to titrate the level of anesthesia to match more closely the degree of stimulation results in greater hemodynamic stability and lower total drug dosage. Also, the tendency of opioid blood levels to oscillate above and below the ideal level is minimized [62, 64, 65].

An understanding of basic pharmacokinetic principles and parameters is essential for using continuous narcotic infusions during coronary artery bypass surgery.

Pharmacokinetic principles

Narcotic loading dose (LD) is calculated from the following equation:

LD = (Vdss) (Cp) (Wt)

where LD is loading dose (µg), Vdss is volume of distribution, steady state (ml/kg), Cp is plasma concentration (ng/ml), and Wt is weight (kg).

Maintenance infusion rate (MIR) is calculated as follows:

MIR = (Cl) (Cp) (Wt)

where MIR is maintenance infusion rate (µg/kg/min), Cl is systemic clearance (ml/kg/min), Cp is plasma concentration (ng/ml), and Wt is weight (kg).

The pharmacokinetic parameters utilized for intravenous infusion anesthesia with fentanyl or sufentanil are listed in table 2-3.

Sprigge et al. observed that a loading dose of 50 mcg/kg and maintenance infusion rate of 0.5 µg/kg/min (infusion terminated during rewarming on bypass or after a total dose of 100 µg/kg) produced a stable fentanyl plasma concentration of 15 ng/ml [60]. When fentanyl plasma concentration was maintained at 15 ng/ml, fewer than 50% of patients experienced tachycardia and hypertension during CABG, and those that did were easily treated with supplemental nitrous oxide, nitroglycerin, droperidol, or volatile anesthetics. This study and others suggest that additional cardiovascular stability may be

Table 2-3. Pharmacokinetic parameters used for intravenous
infusion anesthesia with fentanyl or sufentanil

Agents	Vdss (L/kg)	Cl (ml/kg/min)	Cp (for CABG) (ng/ml)
Fentanyl	4.0	14	15–25
Sufentanil	1.7	13	5–10

achieved by supplementing the induction dose of fentanyl with a continuous intravenous infusion [28, 58]. Intravenous narcotic administration by continuous infusion thus provides another example of the importance of carefully titrating anesthetic dose to clinical effect.

Sufentanil, a new synthetic derivative of fentanyl, has recently become available for clinical use. While pharmacologically similar to fentanyl, sufentanil provides a number of advantages including greater potency (5–10 times more than fentanyl), more effective blockade of hemodynamic and hormonal responses to surgical stimulation, a more rapid onset of action, and less postoperative respiratory depression [21]. Indeed, when compared with fentanyl in equipotent doses during CABG procedures, sufentanil anesthesia was associated with less hypertension and a reduced requirement for supplemental antihypertensive agents [21]. Sufentanil may, therefore, pending additional clinical experience, prove to be the opioid of choice for coronary artery surgery.

Anesthetic effects on endocrine function

Maintenance of hemodynamic stability throughout the perioperative period requires not only the preservation of myocardial function and vascular tone, but perhaps also inhibition of the endocrine "stress" response" to surgical stimulation. The inhalation anesthetics may be used to partially blunt endocrine responses to stress, but their associated myocardial depressant and/or vasodilator effects are poorly tolerated by patients with CAD and cardiac dysfunction [66]. Morphine, in doses of 0.5–3.0 mg/kg, does not consistently block increases in blood pressure, heart rate, and plasma antidiuretic hormone (ADH) levels induced by surgical stress [11, 67]. Higher doses of morphine (8–11 mg/kg) will inhibit the stress response to surgical stimulation, but also cause increased fluid requirements and prolonged respiratory depression [68].

In contrast, the new synthetic opioids (fentanyl, sufentanil, alfentanil) have been shown to be more effective at both maintaining cardiovascular stability and blunting the hormonal response to surgical stress. Stanley et al. [55, 59], using a high-dose fentanyl (71–75 µg/kg) anesthetic technique, studied the effects of surgical stress during CABG on plasma levels of ADH, cortisol, norepinephrine, and epinephrine. These studies showed plasma levels of ADH, norepinephrine, and epinephrine to be remarkably stable from the time of induction until the initiation of cardiopulmonary bypass (CPB), when all were significantly increased. Plasma cortisol remained at or below control values throughout the operative procedure. In high doses, alfentanil (1.2 mg/kg) and sufentanil (13.1 µg/kg) inhibit increases of plasma ADH and growth hormone throughout the operation, including CPB in patients undergoing CABG procedures [69]. It has been suggested that the relative doses of alfentanil and sufentanil employed in this study were greater than the fentanyl doses used in past studies. However, unpublished data cited by de Lange et al. suggest that fentanyl doses of 150–200 µg/kg are unable to blunt the hormonal stress response to CPB.

The inhibition of "stress-evoked" hormones, while of incompletely determined clinical value, has been shown to improve renal function following coronary artery surgery. Kono et al. [12] compared the effects of halothane–N_2O and fentanyl (100 µg/kg)–N_2O on renal function and stress response during CABG. Following sternal skin incision, patients anesthetized with halothane–N_2O showed significantly higher levels of norepinephrine, epinephrine, aldosterone, cortisol, and vasopressin as well as greater decreases in creatinine clearance than did patients anesthetized with fentanyl. With continued surgical stimulation (pre-CPB), stress hormone levels increased in the halothane–N_2O group and creatinine clearance decreased further. In contrast, hormonal response to surgical stimulation was attenuated by high-dose fentanyl and creatinine clearance remained unchanged. Changes in renal function during halothane–N_2O anesthesia were attributed to a maked increase in stress hormone response to surgical stress: thus, the successful inhibition of stress hormone release by fentanyl–N_2O anesthesia may preserve renal function in addition to the maintenance of hemodynamic stability.

Other studies have compared hemodynamic and endocrine responses to surgical stimulation during anesthesia employing the new synthetic opioids or potent volatile anesthetic agents. Zurick et al. [4] compared the hemodynamic and hormonal effects of fentanyl (150 µg/kg) and halothane–N_2O anesthesia during CABG procedures. They found no significant increases in plasma epinephrine, norepinephrine, or renin activity following intubation or sternotomy in either group, and suggested that the preoperative use of propranolol may have been partially responsible for their findings.

Samuelson et al. [7] studied stress hormone responses in patients undergoing CABG with either sufentanil or enflurane–N_2O anesthesia. Sufentanil was initially administered as a bolus of 15 µg/kg for induction of anesthesia; however, declining plasma sufentanil levels resulted in hypertension during CPB. This was treated with an additional dose of 10 µg/kg sufentanil at the onset of CPB. Plasma epinephrine and norepinephrine levels remained at or near control values prior to CPB in the sufentanil groups while a small increase in epinephrine immediately prior to CPB was observed in the enflurane–N_2O group. During CPB, norepinephrine levels were higher in the group receiving sufentanil as a single bolus at the time of induction (no supplementation at CPB) while plasma epinephrine levels were elevated in both the unsupplemented sufentanil group and the enflurane–N_2O group. Blunting of the stress hormone response appears to be best provided by sufentanil when plasma levels are maintained at an adequate level throughout the surgical procedure. This can be accomplished by intermittent bolus or continuous sufentanil infusion [63]. Maintenance of adequate plasma opioid levels throughout the operative procedure may also be an important factor contributing not only to the inhibition of stress hormones, but also to the prevention of hypertension, tachycardia, and intraoperative awareness.

A possible mechanism for the relatively increased levels of stress hormones associated with the use of inhalational anesthetic agents may involve the fluctuation of plasma drug levels during the "peaks and valleys" of surgical stress. Both Zurick et al. [4] and Samuelson et al. [7] report slightly less stable hemodynamics or required "fine tuning" adjustments of the inhalation agent dose in order to facilitate cardiovascular stability during CABG (figure 2-1). This problem should not arise if adequate blood levels of potent narcotics (especially sufentanil) are maintained throughout the surgical procedure.

Supplemental agents

Fentanyl anesthesia for CABG, while quite popular, has not proven to be completely "problem free." Various reports of incidents involving intraoperative tachycardia, hypertension, and recall require careful consideration [20, 70–73]. A variety of supplementary agents have been used with fentanyl in an effort to eliminate these incidents and/or reduce the required dose of fentanyl. Unfortunately, the use of supplements during fentanyl anesthesia may result in some loss of cardiovascular stability. Nitrous oxide, the most common supplement, used in combination with fentanyl increases systemic vascular resistance and decreases cardiac output and blood pressure [58]. Diazepam, in a similar manner, results in cardiovascular depression when administered during, or prior to, fentanyl anesthesia [31]. While other intravenous supplements, such as scopalomine and droperidol, appear not to depress the myocardium when used with fentanyl, their individual properties may prove detrimental. For example, droperidol decreases systemic vascular resistance and mean arterial pressure [74, 75]. This can compromise coronary perfusion pressure. Scopolamine may increase heart rate and/or cause postoperative dysphoria, both of which could adversely affect myocardial oxygen balance [76].

Volatile inhalation agents may prove to be the best supplements for high-dose fentanyl anesthesia. If these agents are to be used successfully as supplements, careful dose titration is essential. Otherwise, fall in mean arterial pressure secondary to myocardial depression and systemic vasodilation is likely. Moffitt et al. observed favorable myocardial oxygenation, metabolism, and hemodynamics when enflurane was used as a supplement to fentanyl (30

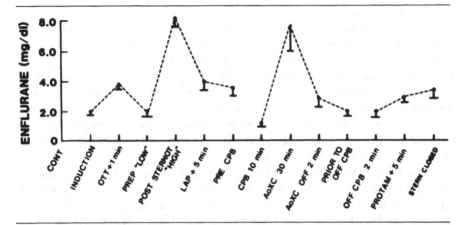

Figure 2-1. Plot of serum enflurane concentrations (mean ± SEM) versus sample time: *CONT*, control/baseline; *INDUCTION*, induction; *OTT + 1 min*, 1 min after orotracheal intubation: *PREP "LOW"*, lowest systolic pressure during prepping; *POST STERNOT "HIGH"*, highest systolic blood pressure after sternotomy; *LAP + 5 min*, 5 min after left artial line placement; *PRE CPB*, preceding cardiopulmonary bypass; *CPB 10 min*, 10 min into cardiopulmonary bypass; *AoXC 30 min*, 30 min after the aortic cross-clamp was placed; *AoXC OFF 2 min*, 2 min after the aortic cross-clamp was removed; *PRIOR TO OFF CPB*, immediately prior to coming off cardiopulmonary bypass; *OFF CPB 2 min*, 2 min after coming off cardiopulmonary bypass; *PROTAM + 5 min*, 5 min after protamine administration; and *STERM CLOSED*, at sternal closure. No significant difference was found between groups. From Samuelson et al. [7].

µg/kg) anesthesia during CABG. Less favorable results were obtained when either fentanyl or inhalation anesthesia was used alone [77].

Neuromuscular blocking agents

Providing neuromuscular blockade for endotracheal intubation and anesthetic maintenance during CABG is yet another source of controversy. A popular approach has been to administer pancuronium as an intravenous bolus (0.1 mg/kg) stimultaneously with a large dose of fentanyl as a bolus or infusion [20, 78]. This method of induction minimizes bradycardia and reduces the incidence of chest wall rigidity; however, the ability to evaluate the patient's level of consciousness and insure an adequate depth of anesthesia is lost [20, 79]. In addition, recent reports have shown that large boluses of pancuronium in combination with fentanyl result in an increased incidence of tachycardia and hypertension in response to laryngoscopy and surgical stimulation. [14, 80] Sonntag et al. observed adverse changes in myocardial blood flow including production of myocardial lactate with the pancuronium bolus–fentanyl infusion technique [80]. A recent study by Thomson and Putnins compared three muscle relaxant regimens—pancuronium, metubine, or pancuronium-metubine combination—in patients undergoing CABG with fentanyl anesthesia administered as a rapid infusion [14]. The authors observed marked increases in heart rate (28%–57%) and a 25% incidence of myocardial ischemia in the group receiving pancuronium alone. No electrocardiographic or heart rate changes were observed in the other two groups. This study provides an illustration of the serious consequences that may result when a large bolus of pancuronium is administered during intravenous induction of anesthesia.

Stanley et al. did not observe ischemic electrocardiographic or heart rate changes despite the use of pancuronium during CABG with fentanyl anesthesia [31, 55, 59]. In these studies, however, succinylcholine was administered for tracheal intubation and pancuronium used for maintenance of neuromuscular blockade. Thus, the timing of pancuronium administration may play an important role in the development of hemodynamic and/or ischemic changes during CABG with fentanyl anesthesia. As with all other agents used to supplement fentanyl anesthesia, neuromuscular blocking agents must be administered cautiously and carefully titrated to clinical effect [78].

Cardiopulmonary bypass

The initiation of cardiopulmonary bypass (CPB) results in several major physiologic perturbations in the patient undergoing CABG [81]. Consequently, the anesthetic management of the patient during this period is unique. This section examines the implications of CPB on intravenous anesthetic techniques for CABG.

The onset of CPB results in hemodilution of the patient's blood volume secondary to the administration of CPB pump-priming solution. Typically, a 40%–50% dilution of plasma occurs and the plasma concentration of drugs will decrease correspondingly [81, 82]. Hypothermia, nonpulsatile perfusion, exclusion of the lungs from circulation, and alterations in protein binding also modify drug kinetics during CPB [81–83]. Lunn et al. [58], Bovill and Sebel [84] and Hug and Molderhaver [62] observed decreases of 37%, 53%, and 42% in plasma fentanyl concentrations immediately following the institution of CPB. After this acute reduction, fentanyl plasma levels remained relatively constant for the remainder of bypass. Koska et al. [82] and Hug [83] reported that CPB prolonged the elimination half-life and clearance of fentanyl, and attributed this effect to the hypothermia and altered hepatic blood flow associated with CPB. In addition, fentanyl is taken up by the lungs to a considerable extent and elimination of the pulmonary system from the circulation during CPB may contribute to the stability of fentanyl plasma levels following their initial decrease after initiation of CPB [85].

There is some controversy as to whether or not it is necessary to restore plasma fentanyl concentration to prebypass levels after the onset of CPB. Since the majority of administered fentanyl is in tissues rather than plasma immediately prior to initiation of CPB, central nervous system drug concentration probably does not change as dramatically as does plasma drug concentration following hemodilution [86]. Furthermore, fentanyl's prolonged elimination half-life during the remainder of CPB and in the immediate postoperative period tends to maintain plasma concentrations at values similar to those occurring shortly after the initiation of CPB [81]. On the other hand, there appears to be a close correlation between plasma fentanyl levels and fentanyl clinical effect [64]. Hug and Moldenhauer demonstrated that, when plasma fentanyl levels decreased to less than 10 ng/ml, patients became responsive to sound and required supplementation with diazepam. When plasma fentanyl levels were maintained at 17 ng/ml or greater via a continuous infusion of 0.3 ng/kg/min, no patient showed signs of responsiveness until 4 h after surgery [62]. Thus, maintaining a continuous infusion of fentanyl from the prebypass period though CPB ensures a steady plasma fentanyl concentration and decreases the likelihood of awareness during coronary artery surgery.

While vast improvements have been made in surgical and bypass techniques, significant postbypass neurologic complications continue to occur. Reported incidence of neuropsychiatric complications following CABG range as high as 40% [87]. Recent data suggest that these neurologic deficits are due to focal, incomplete brain ischemia secondary to intravascular emboli introduced during cannulation of the aorta and right atrium in preparation for bypass or during the surgical procedure itself [87].

Intravenous agents, specifically barbiturates, have been reported to improve neurologic outcome after focal, incomplete brain ischemic episodes in a number of animals studies [88–90]. Recently Nussmeier et al. have shown that sodium thiopental in doses of 25–30 mg/kg protects the human brain when administered prior to the initiation of CPB [91]. The study evaluated patients undergoing open-ventricle procedures at a single institution; therefore, its conclusions may not apply to all patients undergoing coronary artery surgery at other centers employing a variety of anesthetic techniques and CPB protocols. Also, since the cost of barbiturate therapy was an increased requirement for inotropic agents following CPB and prolonged postoperative mechanical ventilation, the recommendations for barbiturate therapy in all patients undergoing bypass require further corroborative study [92].

The potential use of potent inhalational anesthetic agents as a means of brain protection in patients undergoing CABG procedures is limited. While isoflurane has been shown to reduce cerebral oxygen consumption in animals, this effect was observed only at high concentrations (2 MAC), which cause severe and unacceptable cardiovascular depression [93]. Thus, the potential for brain protection with isoflurane or other volatile agents is limited by their cardiovascular depressant effects.

POSTOPERATIVE CONSIDERATIONS

The immediate postoperative period following CABG surgery with high-dose narcotic anesthesia is characterized by continued hemodynamic stability and a high level of analgesia. In contrast, when a primarily inhalation anesthetic technique is used for CABG operations, patients often require significant amounts of analgesics and/or vasodilators for blood pressure stabilization and relief of pain and anxiety [7, 94].

McIlvaine and co-workers reported a 23.7% incidence of hypertension following coronary artery surgery with halogenated agents as the primary anesthetic. However, when high-dose narcotic regimens (morphine 1.0–1.5 mg/kg) were used, the incidence of postoperative hypertension decreased to 2.5% [94]. Samuelson et al. found that significantly greater amounts of sodium nitroprusside were required for control of post-CABG hypertension by patients who were anesthetized were either enflurane–N_2O or a single bolus dose of sufentanil (15 µg/kg) than in patients given 25 µg/kg sufentanil in divided doses [7]. Similarly, morphine requirements for postoperative pain control were significantly less in patients who had received the divided-dose sufentanil regimen.

Benefiel and co-workers recently compared sufentanil with isoflurane anesthesia in patients undergoing aortic reconstruction surgery [95]. A total of 100 patients were randomly assigned to receive either sufentanil or isoflurane for maintenance of anesthesia during the operative procedure. The sufentanil group received 10 µg/kg sufentanil for induction and additional intermittent boluses (25 µg) as well as 60% nitrous oxide for maintenance of anesthesia. In the isoflurane group, anesthesia was induced with thiopental and isolfurane, and maintained with isoflurane. The authors observed significant reductions in the incidence of postoperative renal insufficiency and congestive heart failure with sufentanil anesthesia. Whether these results indicate a protective effect associated with sufentanil or deleterious effects of isoflurane when used as the primary anesthetic agent in patients with atherosclerotic vascular disease remains to be determined.

High-dose narcotic anesthesia is associated with a significant incidence of postoperative respiratory depression. Following CABG, up to 17 h may be required for plasma fentanyl concentrations to decline below the threshold for weaning from mechanical ventilation [29, 84, 96]. Efforts to reverse the respiratory effects of high-dose narcotic anesthesia with naloxone have resulted in hypertension, ventricular arrhythmias, pulmonary edema, and sudden death [96–99]. In addition, naloxone's comparatively short (~60 min) duration of action may result in renarcotization and carbon dioxide retention [100]. Thus, the dangers of narcotic reversal with naloxone in the immediate postoperative period appear to outweigh any potential benefit obtained from early extubation and spontaneous respiration. Early extubation has been shown to reduce cardiopulmonary complications and time spent in the intensive care unit (ICU) following primarily inhalation anesthetic techniques [101, 102]. However, since early extubation following narcotic anesthesia for CABG has not been documented to produce any reduction in ICU time [7] or cardiopulmonary complications [103], a gradual decline in plasma opioid levels appears (at the present time) to provide the most favorable clinical conditions after CABG surgery.

If early extubation is considered necessary for patient management following a CABG procedure where primary narcotic anesthesia has been used, a narcotic agonist–antagonist agent may prove valuable. Nalbuphine, a narcotic agonist–antagonist has been used as an alternative agent for reversal of postoperative respiratory depression [15]. Moldenhauer and co-workers administered nalbuphine (1.5–9.0 mg) following coronary artery surgery for reversal of respiratory depression secondary to high-dose fentanyl anesthesia [16]. In this study, nalbuphine was reported to provide favorable extubating conditions an average of 7.7 after CABG. Following narcotic reversal, no evidence of tachycardia, dysrhythmia, or hemodynamic instability was observed. Renarcotization did occur, however, in several patients 2–3 h after nalbuphine administration. This undesired effect was readily reversed with additional nalbuphine. Pain control was maintained successfully with intermittent doses of nalbuphine (avg, 4.7 mg). These observations demonstrate nalbuphine's utility as a reversal agent for post-CABG respiratory depression as well as its effectiveness as an analgesic. Further investigation to determine the optimal dose range and administration times with define nalbuphine's role in the postoperative period following cardiac surgery.

CONCLUSION

The "controversy" surrounding the selection of various intravenous or inhalation anesthetic agents for coronary artery surgery revolves around the anesthesiologists' goal to utilize the safest, most effective, techniques possible. While the ultimate test of an anesthetic's superiority—perioperative morbidity or "outcome"—has not conclusively shown any agent to be of particular advantage for CABG surgery, the new synthetic opioids provide a hemodynamically stable perioperative environment for patients with varying degrees of cardiovascular dysfunction. Thus, the "controversy" continues as new and better agents and techniques are developed for use in the management of patients during coronary artery surgery.

REFERENCES

1. Roizen MF: Does choice of anesthetic (narcotic versus inhalational) significantly affect cardiovascular outcome after cardiovascular surgery. In: Estatanous FG (ed) Opioids in anesthesia. Butterworth, Boston, 1984, pp 180–189.
2. Conahan III TJ, Ominsky AJ, Wollman H, Stroth RA: A prospective random comparison of halothane and morphine for open-heart anesthesia: one year's experience. Anesthesiology 38:528–535, 1973.
3. Kistner JR, Miller ED Jr, Lake CL, Ross WT Jr: Indices of myocardial oxygenation during coronary-artery revascularization in man with morphine versus halothane anesthesia. Anesthesiology 50:324–330, 1979.

4. Zurick AM, Urzua J, Yared J-P, Estafanous FG: Comparison of hemodynamic and hormonal effects of large single-dose fentanyl anesthesia and halothane/nitrous oxide anesthesia for coronary artery surgery. Anesth Analg 61:521–526, 1982.
5. Moffitt EA, Sethna DH, Bussell JA, Raymond M, Matloff JM, Gray RJ: Myocardial metabolism and hemodynamic responses to halothane or morphine anesthesia for coronary artery surgery. Anesth Analg 61:979–985, 1982.
6. Heikkila H, Jalonen J, Arola M, Laaksonen V: Haemodynamics and myocardial oxygenation for coronary artery surgery: comparison between enflurane and high-dose fentanyl anaesthesia. Acta Anaesthesiol Scand 29:457–464, 1985.
7. Samuelson PN, Reves JG, Kirklin JK, Bradley E Jr, Wilson KD, Adams M: Comparison of sufentanil and enflurane–nitrous oxide anesthesia for myocardial revascularization. Anesth Analg 65:217–226, 1986.
8. Moffitt EA, Sethna DH: The coronary circulation and myocardial oxygenation in coronary artery disease: effects of anesthesia. Anesth Analg 65:395–410, 1986.
9. Roberts SL, Tinker JH: Narcotics versus inhalation anesthetics: effects on regional myocardial ischemia. In: Estatanous FG (ed) Opioids in anesthesia. Butterworth, Boston, 1984, pp 190–193.
10. Milocco I, Lof BA, William-Olsson G, Appelgren LK: Left ventricular function during anaesthesia induction and sternotomy in patients with ischaemic heart disease: a comparison of six anaesthetic techniques. Acta Anaesthesiol Scand 29:241–249, 1985.
11. Philbin DM, Coggins CH: Plasma antidiuretic hormone levels in cardiac surgical patients during morphine and halothane anesthesia. Anesthesiology 49:95–98, 1978.
12. Kono K, Philbin DM, Coggins CH, Moss J, Rosow CE, Schneider RC, Slater EE: Renal function and stress response during halothane or fentanyl anesthesia. Anesth Analg 60:552–556, 1981.
13. Slogoff S, Keats AS: Does perioperative myocardial ischemia lead to postoperative myocardial infarction? Anesthesiology 62:107–114, 1985.
14. Thomson IR, Putnins CL: Adverse effects of pancuronium during high-dose fentanyl anesthesia for coronary artery bypass grafting. Anesthesiology 62:708–713, 1985.
15. Latasch L, Probst S, Dudziak R: Reversal by nalbuphine of respiratory depression caused by fentanyl. Anesth Analg 63:814–816, 1984.
16. Moldenhauer CC, Roach GW, Finlayson DC, Hug CC Jr, Kopel ME, Tobia V, Kelly S: Nalbuphine antagonism of ventilatory depression following high-dose fentanyl anesthesia. Anesthesiology 62:647–650, 1985.
17. Heisterkamp DV, Cohen PJ: The use of naloxone to antagonize large doses of opiates administered during nitrous oxide anesthesia. Anesth Analg 53:12–18, 1974.
18. Kennedy JW, Kaiser GC, Fisher LD, Fritz JK, Myers W, Mudd JG, Ryan TJ: Clinical and angiographic predictors of operative mortality from the collaborative study in coronary artery surgery (CASS). Circulation 63:793–802, 1981.
19. Clark NJ, Stanley TH: Anesthesia for vascular surgery. In: Miller R (ed) Anesthesia, vol 2, 2nd edn. Churchill Livingstone, New York, 1986, ch 42, pp 1519–1562.
20. Bovill JG, Sebel PS, Stanley TH: Opioid analgesics in anesthesia: with special reference to their use in cardiovascular anestheseia. Anesthesiology 61:731–755, 1984.
21. de Lange S, Boscoe MJ, Stanley TH, Pace N: Comparison of sufentanil–O_2 and fentanyl–O_2 for coronary artery surgery. Anesthesiology 56:112–118, 1982.
22. Moffitt EA, Scovil JE, Barker RA, Marble AE, Sullivan JA, DelCamp C, Cousins CL, Kinley CE: Myocardial metabolism and haemodynamic responses during high-dose fentanyl anaesthesia for coronary patients. Can Anaesth Soc J 31:611–618, 1984.
23. Howie MB, McSweeney TD, Lingam RP, Maschke SP: A comparison of fentanyl–O_2 and sufentanil–O_2 for cardiac anesthesia. Anesth Analg 64:877–887, 1985.
24. Moffitt EA, Imrie DD, Scovil JE, Glenn JJ, Cousins CL, DelCamp C, Sullivan JA, Kinley CE: Myocardial metabolism and haemodynamic responses with enflurane anaesthesia for coronary artery surgery. Can Anaesth Soc J 31:604–610, 1984.
25. Moffitt EA, Barker RA, Glenn JJ, Imrie DD, DelCamp C, Landymore RW, Kinley CE, Murphy DA: Myocardial metabolism and hemodynamic responses with isoflurane anesthesia for coronary arterial surgery. Anesth Analg 65:53–61, 1986.
26. Reiz S, Balfors E, Sorensen MB, Ariola S Jr, Friedman A, Truedsson H: Isoflurane: a

powerful coronary vasodilator in patients with coronary artery disease. Anesthesiology 59:91–97, 1983.

27. Reiz S, Ostman M: Regional coronary hemodynamics during isoflurane–nitrous oxide anesthesia in patients with ischemic heart disease. Anesth Analg 64:570–576, 1985.

28. Wynands JE, Wong P, Whalley DG, Sprigge JS, Townsend GE, Patel YC: Oxygen–fentanyl anesthesia in patients with poor left ventricular function: hemodynamics and plasma fentanyl concentrations. Anesth Analg (Cleve) 62:476–482, 1983.

29. Ellison N: Morphine and the new narcotics in postoperative ventilatory control. In: Estafanous FG (ed) Opioids in anesthesia. Butterworth, Boston, 1984, pp 293–296.

30. Stanley TH, de Lange S, Boscoe MJ, de Bruijn N: The influence of chronic preoperative propranolol therapy on cardiovascular dynamics and narcotic requirements during operation in patients with cornary artery disease. Can Anaesth Soc J 29:319–324, 1982.

31. Stanley TH, Webster LR: Anesthetic requirements and cardiovascular effects of fentanyl–oxygen and fentanyl–diazepam–oxygen anesthesia in man. Anesth Analg 57:411–416, 1978.

32. Freis ES, Lappas DG: Chronic administration of calcium entry blockers and the cardiovascular responses to high doses of fentanyl in man. Anesthesiology 57:A295, 1982.

33. Kapur PA: Calcium blockers. In: Estafanous FG (ed) Opioids in anesthesia. Butterworth, Boston, 1984, pp 277–284.

34. Roach GW, Moldenhauer CC, Hug CC Jr, Schultz JD, Curling PE: Hemodynamic responses to fentanyl or diazepam–fentanyl anesthesia in patients on chronic nifedipine therapy. Anesthesiology 61:A374, 1984.

35. Casson WR, Jones RM, Parsons RS: Nifedipine and cardiopulmonary bypass: post-bypass management after continuation or withdrawal of therapy. Anaesthesia 39:1197–1201, 1984.

36. Larach DR, Hensley FA Jr, Pae LR, Ruffle JM, Campbell DB, Pae WE, Pennock JL, Pierce WS: A randomized study of diltiazem withdrawal prior to coronary artery bypass surgery. Anesthesiology 63:A23, 1985.

37. Schick EC Jr, Living C, Heupler FA Jr: Randomized withdrawal from nifedipine: placebo-controlled study in patients with coronary artery spasm. Am Heart J 104:690, 1982.

38. Reves JG, Kissin I, Lell WA, Tosone S: Calcium entry blockers: uses and implications for anesthesiologists. Anesthesiology 57:504–518, 1982.

39. Reves JG: Editorial: the relative hemodynamic effects of Ca^{++} entry blockers. Anesthesiology 61:3–5, 1984.

40. Kates RA, Kaplan JA, Guyton RA, Dorsey L, Hug CC Jr, Hatcher CR: Hemodynamic interactions of verapamil and isoflurane. Anesthesiology. 59:132–138, 1983.

41. Kates RA, Zaggy AP, Norfleet EA, Heath KR: Comparative cardiovascular effects of verapamil, nifedipine and diltiazem during halothane anesthesia in swine. Anesthesiology 61:10–18, 1984.

42. Kapur PA, Bloor BC, Flacke WE, Olewine SK: Comparison of cardiovascular responses to verapamil during enflurane, isoflurane, or halothane anesthesia in the dog. Anesthesiology 61:156–160, 1984.

43. Rogers K, Hysing ES, Merin RG, Taylor A, Hartley C, Chelly JE: Cardiovascular effects of and interaction between calcium blocking drugs and anesthetics in chronically instrumented dogs. II. Verapamil, enflurane, and isoflurane. Anesthesiology 64:568–575, 1986.

44. Campos JH, Kapur PA: Combined effects of verapamil and isoflurane on coronary blood flow and myocardial metabolism in the dog. Anesthesiology 64:778–784, 1986.

45. Kapur PA, Campos JH, Tippit SE: Influence of diltiazem on cardiovascular function and coronary hemodynamics during isoflurane anesthesia in the dog: correlation with plasma diltiazem levels. Anesth Analg 65:81–87, 1986.

46. Marshall AG, Kissin I, Reves JG, Bradley EL Jr, Blackstone EH: Interaction between negative inotropic effects of halothane and nifedipine in the isolated rat heart. J Cardiovasc Pharmacol 5:592–597, 1983.

47. Schulte-Sasse U, Hess W, Markschies-Hornung A, Tarnow J: Combined effects of halothane anesthesia and verapamil on systemic hemodynamics and left ventricular myocardial contractility in patients with ischemic heart disease. Anesth Analg 63:791–798, 1984.

48. Bloor BC, Flacke WE: Reduction in halothane anesthetic requirement by clonidine, an alpha-adrenergic agonist. Anesth Analg 61:741–745, 1982.

49. Wood AJJ: Hypotensive and vasodilator drugs. In: Mandwood AJJ (ed) Drugs and anesthesia. Williams and Wilkins, Baltimore, 1982, pp 447–478.
50. Eger EI, Saidman LJ, Brandstater B: Minimum alveolar anesthetic concentration: a standard of anesthetic potency. Anesthesiology 26:756–763, 1965.
51. Ghignone M, Quintin L, Duke PC, Kehler CH, Calvillo O: Effects of clonidine on narcotic requirements and hemodynamic response during induction of fentanyl anesthesia and endotracheal intubation. Anesthesiology 64:36–42, 1986.
52. Lowenstein E, Hallowell P, Levine FH, Daggett WM, Austin G, Laver MB: Cardiovascular response to large doses of intravenous morphine in man. N Engl J Med 281:1389–1393, 1969.
53. Dalton B: Anaesthesia and coronary heart disease. J Ir Coll Phys Surg 2:36–40, 1972.
54. Stoelting RK, Gibbs PS: Hemodynamic effects of morphine and morphine–nitrous oxide in valvular heart disease and coronary artery disease. Anesthesiology 38:45–52, 1973.
55. Stanley TH, Philbin DM, Coggins CH: Fentanyl–oxygen anaesthesia for coronary artery surgery: cardiovascular and antidiuretic hormone responses. Can Anaesth Soc J 26:168–173, 1979.
56. Stanley TH, de Lange S: The effect of population habits on side effects and narcotic requirements during high-dose fentanyl anesthesia. Can Anaesth Soc J 31:368–376, 1984.
57. Le Lange S, Stanley TH, Boscoe MJ: Fentanyl–oxygen anesthesia: comparison of anesthetic requirements and cardiovascular responses in Salt Lake City, Utah, and Leyden, The Netherlands [abstr]. In: Rugheimer E, Wawersik J, Zindler M (eds) 7th world congress of anaesthesiologists, Hamburg, FRG, 14–21 September 1980. Excerpta Medica, Amsterdam, 1980, p 313.
58. Lunn JK, Stanley TH, Eisele J, Webster L, Woodward A: High dose fentanyl anesthesia for coronary artery surgery: plasma fentanyl concentrations and influence of nitrous oxide on cardiovascular responses. Anesth Analg 58:390–395, 1979.
59. Stanley TH, Berman L, Green O, Robertson D: Plasma catecholamine and cortisol responses to fentanyl–oxygen anesthesia for coronary-artery operations. Anesthesiology 53:250–253, 1980.
60. Sprigge JS, Wynands JE, Whalley DG, Bevan DR, Townsend GE, Nathan H, Patel YC, Srikant CB: Fentanyl infusion anesthesia for aortocoronary bypass surgery: plasma levels and hemodynamic response. Anesth Analg 61:972–978, 1982.
61. Moldenhauer CC, Hug CC: Continuous infusion of fentanyl for cardiac surgery. Anesth Analg 61:206, 1982.
62. Hug CC Jr, Moldenhauer CC: Pharmacokinetics and dynamics of fentanyl infusions in cardiac surgical patients. Anesthesiology 57:A45, 1982.
63. Samuelson PN, Reves JG, Kirklin JK, George J, Bradley EL, Wilson KD, Barker S, Oparil S, Adams ML: Sufentanil infusion anesthesia in patients undergoing valvular heart surgery. Anesthesiology 63:A74, 1985.
64. McClain DA, Hug CC Jr: Intravenous fentanyl kinetics. Clin Pharmacol Ther 28:106–114, 1980.
65. Bovill JG, Sebel PS, Blackburn CL, Oei-Lim V, Heykants JJ: The pharmacokinetics of fentanyl in surgical patients. Anesthesiology 61:502–506, 1984.
66. Flezzani P, Croughwell ND, McIntyre RW, Reves JG: Isoflurane decreases the cortisol response to cardiopulmonary bypass. Anesth Analg 65:1117–1122, 1986.
67. Arens JF, Benbow BP, Ochsner JL, Theard R: Morphine anesthesia for aortocoronary bypass procedures. Anesth Analg 51;901–909, 1972.
68. Stanley TH, Gray NH, Standford W, Armstrong R: The effects of high-dose morphine on fluid and blood requirements in open-heart operations. Anesthesiology 38:536–541, 1973.
69. de Lange S, Boscoe MJ, Stanley TH, de Bruijn N, Philbin DM, Coggins CH: Antidiuretic and growth hormone responses during coronary artery surgery with sufentanil–oxygen and alfentanil–oxygen anesthesia in man. Anesth Analg 61:434–438, 1982.
70. Waller JL, Hug CC Jr, Nagle DM, Craver JM: Hemodynamic changes during fentanyl–oxygen anesthesia for aortocoronary bypass operation. Anesthesiology 55:212–217, 1981.
71. Hilgenberg JC: Intraoperative awareness during high-dose fentanyl–oxygen anesthesia. Anesthesiology 54:341–343, 1981.
72. Mark JB, Greenberg LM: Intraoperative awareness and hypertensive crisis during high-dose

fentanyl–diazepam–oxygen anesthesia. Anesth Analg 62:698–700, 1983.
73. Edde RR: Hemodynamic changes prior to and after sternotomy in patients anesthetized with high-dose fentanyl. Anesthesiology 55:444–446, 1981.
74. Whitwam JG, Russell WJ: The acute cardiovascular changes and adrenergic blockade by droperidol in man. Br J Anaesth 43;581–591, 1971.
75. Dixon SH, Nolan SP, Stewart S, Morrow AG: Neuroleptanalgesia: effects of Innovar[R] on myocardial contractility, total peripheral vascular resistance and capacitance. Anesth Analg 49:331–335, 1970.
76. Bennett GM, Loeser EA, Stanley TH: Cardiovascular effects of scopolamine during morphine–oxygen and morphine–nitrous oxide anesthesia in man. Anesthesiology 46:225–227, 1977.
77. Moffitt EA, McIntyre AJ, Barker RA, Imrie DD, Murphy DA, Landymore RW, Kinley CE: Myocardial metabolism and hemodynamic responses with fentanyl–enflurane anesthesia for coronary arterial surgery. Anesth Analg 65:46–52, 1986.
78. Savarese JJ, Lowenstein E: Editorial: the name of the game—no anesthesia by cookbook. Anesthesiology 62:703–705, 1985.
79. Hill AB, Nahrwold ML, de Rosayro AM, Knight PR, Jones RM, Bolles RE: Prevention of rigidity during fentanyl–oxygen induction of anesthesia. Anesthesiology 55:452–454, 1981.
80. Sonntag H, Larsen R, Hilfiker O, Kettler D, Brockschnieder B: Myocardial blood flow and oxygen consumption during high-dose fentanyl anesthesia in patients with coronary artery disease. Anesthesiology 56:417–422, 1982.
81. Holley FO, Ponganis KV, Stanski DR: Effect of cardiopulmonary bypass on pharmacokinetics of drugs. Clin Pharmacokinet 7:234–251, 1982.
82. Koska AJ, Romagnoli A, Kramer WG: Effect of cardiopulmonary bypass on fentanyl distribution and elimination. Clin Pharmacol Ther 29:100–105, 1981.
83. Hug CC Jr: Pharmacokinetics and dynamics of narcotic analgesics. In: Prys-Roberts C, Hug CC Jr (eds) Pharmacokinetics of anaesthesia. Blackwell, Oxford, 1984, pp 187–234.
84. Bovill JG, Sebel PS: Pharmacokinetics of high-dose fentanyl: study in patients undergoing cardiac surgery. Br J Anaesth 52:795–801, 1980.
85. Bentley JB, Conahan TJ, Cork RC: Fentanyl sequestration in lungs during cardiopulmonary bypass. Clin Pharmacol Ther 34:703–706, 1983.
86. Hug CC Jr, Murphy MR: Tissue redistribution of fentanyl and termination of its effects in rats. Anesthesiology 55:369–375, 1981.
87. Slogoff S, Girgis KZ, Keats AS: Etiologic factors in neuropsychiatric complications associated with cardiopulmonary bypass. Anesth Analg 61:903–911, 1982.
88. Smith AL, Hoff JT, Nielsen SL, Carson CP: Barbiturate protection in acute focal cerebral ischemia. Stroke 5:127, 1974.
89. Michenfelder JD, Milde JH: Influence of anesthetics on metabolic, functional and pathologic responses to regional cerebral ischemia. Stroke 6:405–410, 1975.
90. Michenfelder JD, Milde JH, Sundt TM Jr: Cerebral protection by barbiturate anethesia. Arch Neurol 33:345–350, 1976.
91. Nussmeier NA, Arlund C, Slogoff S: Neuropsychiatric complications after cardiopulmonary bypass: cerebral protection by a barbiturate. Anesthesiology 64:165–170, 1986.
92. Michenfelder JD: Editorial: a valid demonstration of barbiturate-induced brain protection in man—at last. Anesthesiology 64:140–142, 1986.
93. Newberg LA, Milde JH, Michenfelder JD: Systemic and cerebral effects of isoflurane induced hypotension in dogs. Anesthesiology 60:541–546, 1984.
94. McIlvaine W, Boulanger M, Maille JG, Paiement B, Taillefer J, Sahab P: Hypertension following coronary artery bypass graft. Can Anaesth Soc J 29:212–217, 1982.
95. Benefiel DJ, Roizen MF, Lampe GH, Sohn YJ, Fong KS, Irwin DH, Drasner K, Smith JS, Stoney RJ, Ehrenfeld WK, Goldstone JS, Reilly LM, Thisted RA, Eger II EI: Morbidity after aortic surgery with sufentanil vs isoflurane anesthesia. Anesthesiology 65:A516, 1986.
96. Howie MB: Postoperative opioid reversal and analgesia after open heart surgery. In: Estatanous FG (ed) Opioids in anesthesia. Butterworth, Boston, 1984, pp 302–305.
97. Desmonts JM, Bohm G, Couderc E: Hemodynamic responses to low doses of naloxone after narcotic–nitrous oxide anesthesia. Anesthesiology 49:12–16, 1978.
98. Flacke JW, Flacke WE, Williams GD: Acute pulmonary edema following naloxone reversal of high-dose morphine anesthesia. Anesthesiology 47:376–378, 1977.

99. Andree RA: Sudden death following naloxone administration. Anesth Analg 59:782–784, 1980.
100. Smith TC: Opioid reversal and postoperative narcotic analgesia. In: Estafanous FG (ed) Opioids in anesthesia. Butterworth, Boston, 1984, pp 297–301.
101. Klineberg PL, Geer RT, Hirsh RA, Aukburg SJ: Early extubation after coronary artery bypass graft surgery. Crit Care Med 5:272–274, 1977.
102. Quasha AL, Loeber N, Feeley TW, Ullyot DJ, Roizen MF: Postoperative respiratory care: a controlled trial of early and late extubation following coronary-artery bypass grafting. Anesthesiology 52:135–141, 1980.
103. Prakash O, Jonson B, Meij S, Bos E, Hugenholtz PG, Nauta J, Hekman W; Criteria for early extubation after intracardiac surgery in adults. Anesth Analg 56:703–708, 1977.

3. BLOOD GAS VALUES SHOULD BE CORRECTED FOR BODY TEMPERATURE DURING HYPOTHERMIA

ENRICO M. CAMPORESI
RICHARD E. MOON

Widespread clinical application of hypothermia during cardiac surgery has led in recent years to a controversy regarding temperature correction of arterial blood gas values during the management of patients at body temperatures lower than normal.

Early clinical studies on the subject were empirical compilations of outcome in a difficult and developing clinical field. Quite independently, however, biologists were assembling observations on the regulation of body-fluid composition in animals commonly living at diverse body temperatures (poikilotherms) and in mammals during hiberation, leading to solid conceptual frames of great intellectual strength. These various bodies of knowledge have been slowly assimilated during the last few years, but the arguments have not been exhausted upon the interpretation of blood gases from patients maintained at a body temperature different from 37°C, the temperature at which measuring electrodes are maintained. In this chapter, we defend the side of the argument in favor of "correction" of arterial blood gas values for body temperature. During the last few years, this side of the argument has been rapidly losing favor among clinicians who in larger numbers are embracing the opposing view of non-correcting blood gas values, on the strength on the experimental evidence that anaerobic cooling (and warming) of blood samples follows the rule of *constant alkalinity*. Little compelling new evidence is available or forthcoming in favor of correction. However, on critical analysis, the argument in favor of correction can be supported and is accompanied by good clinical results.

DEFINITIONS

The clinical value of reducing the normal body temperature in patients during anesthesia to hypothermic levels is based on the associated decreased rate of cellular reactions and the attendant reduction in oxygen dependence of the affected organs. This is often the choice during cardiopulmonary bypass in order to protect the ischemic myocardium and with the scope of preserving function to other organs of the body, especially the brain, when perfusion may be limited. The problem of interpretation of blood gases obtained at a body temperature well below 37°C is the following: all blood gas analyzers are temperature sensitive, and the measurement is obtained with electrodes thermostated at 37°C. The interpretation of blood gas values measured at 37°C can vary if the results obtained at 37°C are used as such (= noncorrected) or if a manual or automatic correction is performed, transforming the data to the temperature of the patient (= corrected) with the aid of a nomogram of fixed constants.

Different considerations apply to the interpretation of values for Pao_2 than for both pH and $Paco_2$. This is discussed later in the chapter.

The traditional view of anesthesiologists [1] was to adjust arterial blood Pco_2 (e.g., add a stream of CO_2 to the oxygenator on cardiopulmonary bypass during hypothermia) in order to adjust the pH of the blood at the patient's temperature to 7.42. This is the view in favor of "correcting" pH and Pco_2 for body temperature, or in favor of maintaining a constant pH value at the patient body temperature. This strategy has also been named *pH-stat*. In recent years, a new opinion has emerged, based on the principle popularized by Rahn et al. [2] that the proper reference value to be defended at all temperatures may be electrochemical neurality within the cell. With cooling, the pH of the neutral point of water rises, and neutrality shifts toward more alkaline pH values. Since the measured pH obtained at an electrode temperature of 37°C is equal to 7.40, this system is equivalent to noncorrecting for temperature. Studies on several vertebrate species (frog, turtle) living at different body temperatures (heterotherms or poikilotherms) are consistent with this interpretation [3]. Since the core of this interpretation is based on the fact that the alpha–imidazole chain of blood (and tissue) proteins is the principal buffer system at all body temperatures, this management strategy has also been named *alpha-stat*.

Recent observations on a different type of natural experiment, namely, the hibernating mammal, which lives for long periods at low body temperatures, have shown that pH and Pco_2 are actively regulated during cold survival (CO_2 accumulates and corrected pH is close to 7.4). It has been suggested that imitation of the hibernating mammal is a more appropriate response for a homeotherm such as man during body cooling [4], rather than following the example of the cold frog.

HEMODILUTION AND HYPOTHERMIA

Clinical practice for over two decades has demonstrated the usefulness of utilizing two adjunct treatments during cardiopulmonary bypass: hemodilution and hypothermia. Hemodilution produces several advantages, starting with reduction of the need for donated blood, or blood products, with attendant reduced risks of transfusion. The reduction in hematocrit also reduces blood viscosity and plasma proteins, as well as red-cell content, at a time when hypothermia would otherwise increase flow resistance of undiluted blood in peripheral vascular beds [5, 6]. The reduction in viscosity achieved with hemodilution will allow a given flow to be achieved with lower perfusion pressures [7]. This consideration applies to all vascular beds, including the cerebral vascular bed. Autoregulation of cerebral vascular beds appears operative in some experimental studies, causing cerebral blood flow to increase in response to hemodilution [8]. Human studies have also shown a progressive increase in cerebral blood flow with hemodilution [9].

One of the major effects of hypothermia is a reduction in the metabolic rate of tissues. For the brain, this reduction amounts to ~5% per degree of cooling. The concomitant reduction in requirements for tissues is probably the basis for the preservation effect of hypothermia [10, 11]. Information on side effects is variable. Various data from laboratory experiments in cats, dogs, and monkeys have indicated that hypothermia prolonged for hours results in irreversible cerebral effects [6]. However, clinical and experimental results in monkeys show no occurrence of adverse effects after many hours of moderate hypothermia. Even with very deep hypothermia (5°–8°C), White [12] reported no evidence of neurologic sequelae in primates after 1 h of circulatory arrest.

In summary, the extensive experimental and clinical experience accumulated supports that moderate hypothermia (28°C) in conjunction with hemodilution and adequate perfusion pressure (at least 50 mmHg) offers a highly desirable and safe level of cerebral protection. This regimen is utilized extensively during adult cardiopulmonary bypass procedures for a large variety of surgical interventions.

PROBLEMS OF TEMPERATURE MEASUREMENT

While the principle of hypothermia is conceptually simple, a clear-cut definition of the degree of body cooling and of the concept of *body core* can only be arbitrary [13]. It is well known that different body locations reveal measurements of diverse temperatures and in clinical practice several different sites of temperature measurement are commonly used. The most frequently used monitoring sites in cardiac surgical patients are the esophageal, the rectal, and the pulmonary artery. Less frequently used are urinary bladder temperature and the temperature in the auditory meatus, which probably more closely reflects changes in cerebral temperature. Other temperature-reading locations during cardiopulmonary bypass include the arterial inflow line, the venous return pool, and the cardioplegic reservoir temperature. Thus, since different organs are cooled and rewarmed at different rates, the appropriate choice of *correction temperature* should be organ specific. In clinical practice, the esophageal or the pulmonary artery location is used to reflect overall core temperature. It has been shown [14] that esophageal temperatures or pulmonary artery sites provide a rapidly responding site to alteration of central venous temperatures. Compared to rectal temperature, both locations track more readily the rapidly changing values during the cooling phase. It is noticeable that, during active cooling, esophageal temperature reductions precede changes in brain temperature. The cooling period is a more dangerous phase than the warming period since it may be possible at this time to reduce brain perfusion too soon under the mistaken assumption that neural tissues are as cold as the temperatures recorded in the esophagus.

During pump-induced rewarming, again esophageal temperatures lead both rectal or brain temperatures. It is common clinical practice to utilize a difference between esophageal and rectal temperature to indicate incomplete rewarming [15]. Noback and Tinker [16] postulated that, during hypothermia, vasoconstriction is induced, resembling a state of shock. During the warming phase, many vascular beds may fail to dilate for a long time. These temperature gradients persist in the operating room independently of the prevalent type of anesthetic used, halothane or fentanyl [17], suggesting that anesthetic agents themselves do not play a primary role in this phenomenon.

Ross et al. [18] suggested that the relatively rapid increase in central temperature in the operating room may be the result of the body's inability to lose heat due to surface vasoconstriction. It appears that large areas of the body, like the muscle mass, may remain relatively cold for several hours after forced rewarming. This has been clearly demonstrated by Sladen [19] in patients after cardiopulmonary bypass who required an average of 8 h after admission to the intensive care unit to raise rectal temperature from 34.7°C (on admission) to 38.3°C. These observations are important, since they reaffirm the need to evaluate critically the temperature value for which blood gases may be corrected at different times during induced hypothermia.

TEMPERATURE CORRECTION OF O_2 TENSION

If the temperature of a gas-tight syringe of blood is altered, two effects occur. First, the solubility of O_2 in plasma changes. As temperature increases, solubility diminishes [20]. Second, the hemoglobin–O_2 dissociation curve shifts such that hemoglobin binds O_2 less avidly at higher temperatures and vice versa [21]. Both of these effects will result in higher Po_2 after a temperature increase. At low values of O_2 saturation, both effects are present, whereas the former effect is predominant when hemoglobin is fully saturated. Correction algorithms have been formulated [22–25]. The correction algorithm for blood gas machines used clinically is based upon tentative standards produced by the National Committee for Clinical Laboratory Standards [26]. The per-

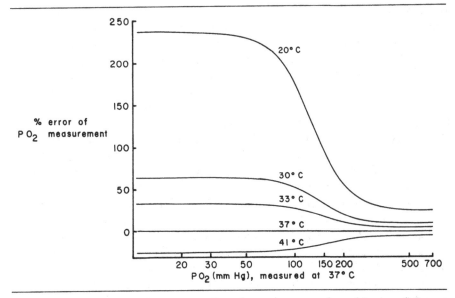

Figure 3-1. Error in Pa_{O_2} measurement expressed as a percentage of actual (corrected) Pa_{O_2} at various body temperatures. Uncorrected Pa_{O_2} is on the abscissa. Percent error is calculated as (P_{O_2} uncorrected − P_{O_2} corrected)/Pa_{O_2} corrected. At low Pa_{O_2} (<30 mmHg), the percent error asymptotically approaches a constant value, determined by hemoglobin–O_2 binding effects. At high Pa_{O_2} (>300 mmHg), O_2 solubility in plasma dominates; thus, the percent error approaches a different asymptote. At temperatures below 37°C the uncorrected P_{O_2} overestimates the actual P_{O_2} (up to 250% at 20°C), whereas above 37°C the uncorrected P_{O_2} is falsely low. In the more common range of temperatures (33°–41°C), the error is less than 35%.

cent error in P_{O_2} measurement at different body temperatures, with the electrode at 37°C, is shown in figure 3-1. The error is largest at low P_{O_2}; therefore, venous P_{O_2} measurements are especially vulnerable to this error. $P\bar{v}_{O_2}$ may be overestimated by nearly 250%, at 20°C.

Despite the considerable controversy regarding temperature correction of pH, there has been little interest in the issue of P_{O_2} correction. In one respect, the argument is an artificial one. A blood sample is drawn at one temperature (body temperature). Measurement of P_{O_2} at another temperature (usually 37°C) will result in a value that is partly a laboratory artifact. The true partial pressure, which will predict physical and chemical activity, and which the organism transduces, is the corrected value. It seems somewhat irrational to use uncorrected values that are in this sense false. The real question, however, is: what is an appropriate P_{O_2} at any given temperature for adequate homeostasis? Put in another way, using some appropriate threshold P_{O_2}, which of the two values obtainable from the blood gas machine ("uncorrected" or "corrected") comes closest to assuring that adequate oxygenation is provided?

Continuous oxygen availability is primarily dependent on perfusion of tissues, oxygen content in blood, and local distribution of flow. Oxygen content in blood at 37°C depends mainly on hemoglobin concentration, but, at lower temperatures, solubility in plasma increases and total tissue demands might be eventually met to a greater degree by dissolved oxygen. In these circumstances, flow may be a critical consideration since, during cardiopulmonary bypass, flow is reduced in order to reduce trauma to blood elements. Hematocrit is simultaneously reduced to decrease sludging in capillaries.

In order to answer the question of correction of Po_2, one must consider various chemical and physiological effects. Since, in clinical practice, the largest changes in temperature occur in the hypothermic range (i.e., less than 37°C) we will confine most of our discussion to those temperatures. However, the issue is also applicable to temperatures above 37°C. As blood is cooled, the two major effects on oxygen–combining capacity must be taken into account. The increase in affinity of hemoglobin for O_2 is commonly known as the *shift to the left*. The most convenient way of expressing this is a decrease in the Po_2 at which hemoglobin is 50% saturated (P_{50}). Figure 3-2 shows the variation in P_{50}, as well as P_{95} and P_{85} (Po_2 values at which hemoglobin is 95% and 85% saturated, respectively), as a function of temperature. The second effect, a change in solubility of O_2 in plasma, results in minor changes in O_2 content that may be significant in the presence of severe anemia. Preliminary analysis would therefore suggest that a lower Po_2 might be tolerable during hypothermia compared to normothermia since hemoglobin binds more O_2 for a given Po_2 and dissolved O_2 in plasma is also increased. The increased solubility of O_2 in plasma is usually clinically insignificant since the percentage of O_2 transported dissolved in plasma is usually less than 5% of the total.

In order to maintain adequate tissue oxygenation, O_2 delivery must be adequate for the tissue O_2 uptake ($\dot{V}o_2$). Whole body $\dot{V}o_2$ has been measured as a function of body temperature (T) in dogs [27]. These investigators found a relationship of the form:

$$\log_{10} \dot{V}o_2 = 0.037 \, T - 0.693 \tag{1}$$

If this equation is applicable to humans, it would predict a decrease in $\dot{V}o_2$ to 23% of control if body temperature is lowered from 37°C to 20°C. Measurements of cerebral O_2 comsumption ($CMRo_2$) have shown a linear relationship with temperature [28], but a decrease of about the same magnitude as whole body $\dot{V}o_2$ at 20°C. Murkin et al. [29] measured $CMRo_2$ in humans, noting a decrease to ~40% of control at 26.5°C, exactly in keeping with equation 1. O_2 delivery is a function of both O_2 content of the blood and blood flow. The effects of temperature on arterial O_2 content are easy to discern from a knowledge of the temperature-related changes in hemoglobin–O_2 affinity. If one is aiming for an O_2 saturation of hemoglobin of 95%, a value that provides a sufficient reserve of safety at 37°C, the required Po_2 will vary from ~100 mmHg at 41°C down to 32 mmHg at 20°C (see figure 3-2), because of the leftward shift of the hemoglobin–O_2 dissociation curve. The corresponding uncorrected Po_2 values are 76 and 93 mmHg, respectively. Therefore, although the corrected Po_2 may be allowed to drop, in fact the uncorrected Po_2 must in-

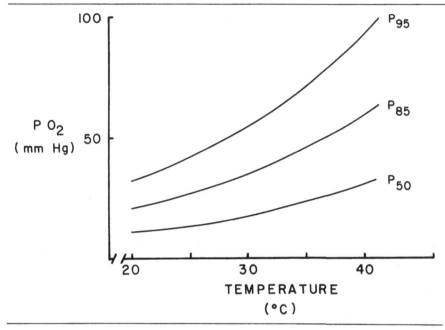

Figure 3-2. Changes in P_{50}, P_{85}, and P_{95} with temperature, calculated for pH = 7.40, corrected to the various temperatures. P_{95}, a PaO_2 usually considered clinically safe, decreases sharply as temperature is lowered from 37°C.

crease as body temperature is lowered. A slightly different and even lower value for PaO_2 may be used if one chooses to maintain uncorrected arterial pH values at 7.40. For example, at 20°C at uncorrected pH of 7.40, a PaO_2 of 24 Torr would maintain 95% saturation of hemoglobin. This is shown in figure 3-3.

There exists another issue, related to local distribution of blood flow. In the capillary, the Po_2 will vary from the arterial value at the proximal end to the venous value as the blood exits. O_2 will diffuse from the capillary blood to the interior of the cell where it is utilized. The simplistic diagram of this process is shown in figure 3-4 in which O_2 flux across the *diffusion resistance* is maintained by the Po_2 gradient from capillary to the mitochondrion. Diffusion resistance is characterized by the physicochemical characteristics of the tissue and the distance required to diffuse (maximally r_D in figure 3-4). If blood flow increases from basal rate, capillaries may be recruited, resulting in higher capillary density and a net decrease in diffusion distance [30]. In contrast, during hypothermia, the decrease in blood flow that occurs may result not only from a decrease in blood flow in individual capillaries but also from total cessation of blood flow in selected blood vessels [31]. This *derecruitment* of capillaries may therefore result in increased diffusion distance. In figure 3-4, the maximum diffusion distance has increased from r_D to r_D'. Thus it appears

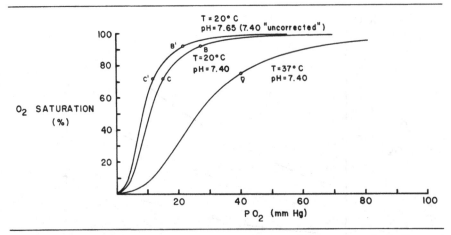

Figure 3-3. Hemoglobin–O_2 dissociation curve as a function of temperature and pH. The usual venous point at 37°C is indicated by $\bar{V}$. At 20°C, B or C represent the venous point, assuming a perfusion flow of 6 L/min or 2 L/min, respectively. Oxygen consumption is scaled to the proper temperature according to equation 1 in the text. Hb concentration is assumed to be 7 g/d. B' and C' are the corresponding venous points if a pH of 7.65 (7.40 "uncorrected") is maintained. The use of uncorrected pH will result in a substantial decrease in venous Po_2 (e.g., 11.5 mmHg at a blood flow of 2 L/min), and hence a possible impairment of diffusion at the tissue level despite what appears to be an adequate $S\bar{v}o_2$.

that, under conditions of sufficiently low capillary Po_2 and blood flow, tissue oxygenation may become limited by diffusion of O_2.

At present, the best indirect assessment of tissue oxygenation is venous Po_2. At 37°C, mixed venous Po_2 is usually around 40 mmHg. At 20°C, a Pao_2 of 32 mmHg will provide adequate arterial O_2 content. However, this must result in a lower venous Po_2 (see figure 3-3). Assuming Vo_2 varies according to equation 1, figure 3-5 delineates the relationship between $P\bar{v}o_2$ and body temperature. The calculations have been made for different blood flows assuming constant arterial Po_2 (corrected to body temperature as well as uncorrected). It is apparent that, at the same total blood flow rate and $\dot{V}o_2$, $P\bar{v}o_2$ is lower for a given uncorrected Pao_2 than for an equivalent corrected value. At 6L/min blood flow, this decrease may be as much as 25%.

These low values of $P\bar{v}o_2$ might theoretically be adequate if $\dot{V}o_2$ decreases with temperature in proportion to the $P\bar{v}o_2$. In other words, if the rate at which O_2 is consumed by a mitochondrion decreases at least as fast as the diffusion gradient from capillary to mitochondrion, then O_2 transport from the capillary into the tissue will occur at a sufficient rate. On the other hand, if the diffusion gradient decreases faster than $\dot{V}o_2$, then diffusion of O_2 to the mitochondrion may limit O_2 utilization. Indeed, $\dot{V}o_2$ decreases to ~25% of basal level as temperature changes from 37°C to 20°C [27], which is roughly proportional to the drop in Pao_2 to 38% of control (100 mmHg to 32 mmHg), and the drop in $P\bar{v}o_2$ (40 to about 15–25 mmHg, depending on pH, Hb, and

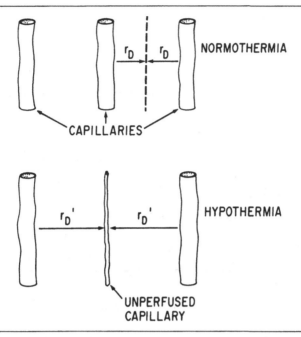

Figure 3-4. The effect of selective underperfusion on capillary-to-mitochondrion diffusion distance. During normothermia, the maximum diffusion distance for O_2 is r_D. During hypothermia, selected capillaries may be unperfused, resulting in a net increase of maximum diffusion distance ($r_{D'}$). This increase in diffusion distance cannot readily be compensated for by an increase in blood flow. Moreover, in clinical practice, blood flow is usually reduced during hypothermia, thereby increasing the risk of tissue hypoxia. This may be more likely if uncorrected Pao_2 values are utilized.

blood flow). This suggests that lower capillary Po_2 may be tolerable at low temperatures. However, this reasoning is only applicable if diffusion distance remains constant; that is, if the distance that the O_2 molecules must diffuse increases while the Po_2 gradient decreases, then rate of diffusion may decrease out of proportion to the change in mitochondrial O_2 consumption. Indeed, diffusion distance may actually increase in hypothermia as already noted, possibly resulting in cellular hypoxia. This is less likely to occur with constant corrected Pao_2 because of the resulting higher $P\bar{v}o_2$. If, instead of assuming an adequate $P\bar{v}o_2$, the clinician chooses to monitor it and adjust Pao_2 and blood flow to obtain a desired value, corrected Po_2 is again preferable. Large errors of overestimation may occur if uncorrected values are used (figure 3-1).

It should be pointed out that, in the event of such diffusion limitation, the venous Po_2 will overestimate tissue Po_2 and hence adequacy of tissue oxygenation. Therefore it seems prudent to maintain Pao_2 at levels that will not only maintain adequate arterial O_2 content but also an adequate diffusion gradient to prevent tissue hypoxia in the event of increased diffusion distance. This may

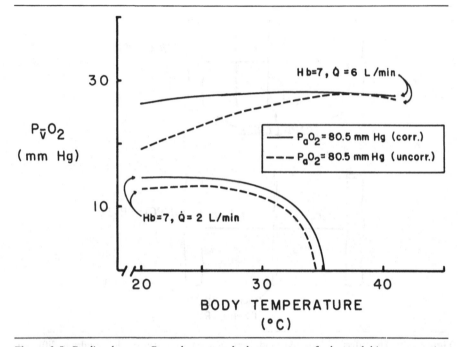

Figure 3-5. Predicted venous Po_2 values versus body temperature for hemoglobin concentration of 7 g/dl, using either corrected or uncorrected $Pao_2 = 80.5$ mmHg, a value that will result in 95% hemoglobin saturation at 37°C. Oxygen consumption is assumed to be 250 ml/min at 37°C, and to decrease with temperature according to equation 1 (see the text). Values are calculated for two extremes of blood flow. In the hypothermic range, even with high flows, $P\bar{v}o_2$ is lower when uncorrected Pao_2 is used: at 20°C the use of corrected Pao_2 will allow $P\bar{v}o_2$ to increase by ~7 mmHg. The curves will vary somewhat depending upon the shape and position of the Hb–O_2 dissociation curve, the temperature correction coefficients, and the effect of temperature on oxygen consumption. However, the essential characteristics will remain the same, provided reasonable assumptions are made for these variables.

best be attained by assessing corrected Po_2 measurements in order not to be lulled into a false sense of security by artificially elevated values.

Parenthetically it should be noted that venous O_2 saturation ($S\bar{v}o_2$) is not particularly useful in this setting. Inspection of figure 3-3 will reveal that $S\bar{v}o_2$ may be extremely high during hypothermia, providing no obvious warning of possible tissue hypoxia.

We must emphasize that we are proposing a conservative viewpoint only on the basis of reasonable speculation until more definitive measures of cellular oxygenation, such as near-infrared absorption to assess cytochrome redox state [32], can either confirm or refute this hypothesis.

We conclude that, despite the difficulties in defining *body temperature*, the use of uncorrected Po_2 values is unsafe. One obtains a false sense of security by maintaining uncorrected Po_2 at some value arbitrarily considered safe at 37°C, since this may lead to a potentially dangerous decrease in the O_2 diffusion gradient at the tissue.

Similar considerations may be applied to the issue of PCO_2 correction. However, a more central issue is the effect of temperature on pH, which is partly determined by the partial pressure of CO_2. Due to the relatively linear CO_2 dissociation curve, adequate CO_2 transport can continue over a wide range of PCO_2 values. Thus, the absolute value for PCO_2 is less important directly than its effect on pH.

THE CONCEPT OF ALPHA-STAT

Even during normothermia, when core temperature is normally maintained at 37°C, not all regions of the body are kept at this temperature level. Large regional differences exist in man such that tissue cells and blood operate normally at temperatures substantially different from 37°C. In a recent review, Reeves [33] concludes that the body does not appear to protect pH as temperature changes, but possibly other properties like the degree of protein ionization.

In a closed system, such as the blood leaving the heart at 37°C and perfusing a colder extremity, the pH of arterial blood increases by 0.015 units for each °C of cooling. The partial pressure of CO_2 decreases nonlinearly as solubility is increased at lower temperatures. If a blood sample is considered while traveling from the heart (at 37°C) to the capillaries in a hand at 7°C, pH (noncorrected) increases from 7.4 to 7.9 units, and $PaCO_2$ decreases from 40 to 10 mmHg, while the CO_2 content is maintained constant. Similar and opposite changes in values have been reported within exercising muscles when local temperature is raised to 42°C (pH 7.35 and PCO_2 47 mmHg, respectively) [34]. The salient feature of this type of analysis has been to recognize that *normal* acid–base status requires a different set of pH and $PaCO_2$ values at each temperature and that oscillations in both directions may indeed be large, and do not induce irreversible alterations in the body. These changes are in fact commonly experienced during normal active life. The slope of the pH-temperature relationship of blood in vitro has been satisfactorily explained [35] by the simultaneous presence and interaction of two buffer systems in blood, one being the carbonic acid–bicarbonate system and the other being an imidazole derivative, namely, the protein-bound–free histidine system. The concentration of protein-bound imidazole groups in blood can account largely for the parallelism between the temperature-dependent pH of blood and that of pure H_2O. An illustration of these relationships at various temperatures for anaerobically cooled human blood and for several animal models is shown in figure 3-6. This illustration summarizes the ubiquitous poikilothermic response to lower body temperature, which provides *constant alkalinity*, in comparison to the neutrality line of water (pNH_2O in figure 3-6). This maintained parallelism has been interpreted as useful to body homeostasis for a variety of reasons. The

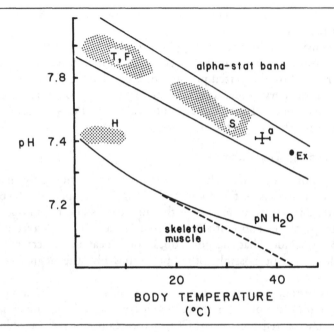

Figure 3-6. pH values recorded at various body temperatures: *a* indicates the range of resting human values *Ex* represents blood values during exercise in a warm muscle, and *S* indicates values for blood perfusing skin at lower temperatures. *T,F* is the range observed in turtles and frogs (poikilotherms) during cold exposure. The *band* surrounding these points defines the range of values utilized when pH is noncorrected, corresponding to the alpha-stat strategy during cardiopulmonary bypass. The *cloud* defined by *H* summarizes the region of arterial pH measured in hibernators. The *line* PNH$_2$O describes the dissociation of pure water, while the *interrupted line* below defines values observed intracellularly in skeletal muscle preparations.

alpha-stat regimen preserves the ratio of [OH$^-$] ions to [H$^+$] ions in blood, conserves protein ionization level, maintains enzyme reactivity optimal at lower temperatures, and preserves Donnan-equilibrium-dependent gradients across cell membranes, such as a constant volume of erythrocytes at all temperatures [36].

The utilization of this strategy (noncorrection) has been also shown to produce beneficial results in experimental preparations in vivo. Strong evidence has documented a favorable effect of relative alkalosis on cardiac contractility [37], on hypothermic ventricular fibrillation threshold [38], an improvement of total left ventricular coronary flow [39] and, more importantly, an increase in the speed of recovery of contractility after a period of prolonged ischemia. A complete summary of more recent experiences has been published [40]. Among the experimentalists, these authors suggest a regimen proposing even more profound alkalosis during hypothermia (rather than just the "relative alkalosis" of noncorrection), on the strength of the more rapid return of left ventricular function observed with a "noncorrection" strategy. The weight of the evidence is clearly that myocardial contractility is superior at temperatures between 26° and 30°C when pH of perfusing blood ranges between 7.7 and 8.1 (or is maintained to 7.4 at 37°C, uncorrected). Despite this trend, which has slowly convinced most cardiac surgical teams to adopt a philosophy of non-correcting pH for temperature, a large group of mammals, the hibernators, adopts with large success a different strategy (pH-stat) for survival at very low temperatures, for very long periods of time.

PHYSIOLOGY OF HIBERNATION

The response of hibernators to prolonged and reversible lowering of body temperature is markedly different from the response of poikilotherm vertebrates and it supports the theory of *correcting* blood gas values to the temperature of the cold body after measuring the values at 37°C. This *constant pH* strategy involves loading considerable amounts of CO_2 during the entrance into hibernation, and hyperventilating to eliminate this CO_2 during the arousal and warming phase. Since most experimental observations have demonstrated a simultaneous reduction in blood concentration of alpha-imidazole, the interpretation of blood gases during hibernation hypothermia is commonly one of respiratory acidosis during the reduction in body temperature [41]. The respiratory acidosis, however, is not equally distributed throughout the body, since it appears that at least two organs, the heart and the liver, show evidence of some metabolic compensation and their acid–base status more properly falls on the alpha–stat curve. There is experimental evidence of a maintained constant alpha–imidazole concentration in extracts from these organs. It is therefore suggestive that the respiratory acidosis may exert inhibitory effects on metabolism, and on nervous tissues in particular. During arousal phases, hyperventilation and correction of intracellular acidosis precede the increase in body temperature. Total oxygen consumption peaks during rewarming at the time of most rapid increase in temperature, preceding the final adjustment toward the temperature plateau of the awake state.

Hibernation in higher-order mammals is apparently a physiological phenomenon that differs in several ways from the survival at low body temperature of poikilotherms, such as frogs and toads. The phenomenon has been reported in several orders of mammals from the primitive echidna to small primates. The best-studied group comprises rodents, such as marmots, squirrels, and bats. Typically the mammal entering hibernation at the beginning of winter chooses a secluded spot after storing large quantities of body fat and actively reduces body temperature, from 37°C to as low as 3°C, for one to several weeks at a time, alternating the cold periods with short arousal periods. During arousal, the animal spontaneously rewarms back to 37°C in very few hours, stays normothermic for several hours, and then returns to hibernation. Oxygen consumption during the cold periods can be reduced 30 times from normothermic metabolic rates [42]. The energy savings expected by the survival at low temperature approximates 97% of the expenditure at normal temperature, a remarkably high saving rate, only somewhat reduced by the expenditure of periodic arousal, which represents over 80% of the total energy used during hibernation. Even though metabolic activity is deeply reduced during hibernation, it is not completely suppressed: circulation and ventilation are kept operative at very low temperatures. Higher cortical activity is generally inhibited, with only evoked potentials being visible on the otherwise flat cortical EEG [43], but brainstem activity is maintained. Other adaptation processes are present, with replacement of enzymes present in the summer with isoenzymes with nearly constant affinity for substrate at lower temperatures.

A significant difference of the hibernator from the ectothermic vertebrate is that most ectotherms can only increase metabolic rate five or six times above the basal level at any given temperature, while hibernators can vary oxygen consumption up to a factor of 40 times at the same body temperature (e.g., 18°C), depending on whether this body temperature is reached during arousal or induction of hibernation. It is suggestive that the ability to inhibit or to increase metabolism so rapidly is a distinctive feature that must require an active metabolic depression. This metabolism-inhibiting factor has been often suggested to be linked with the elevated CO_2 concentration in blood, leading to the respiratory acidosis.

THE CONSTANT PH DURING HIBERNATION

Arterial blood pH and P_{CO_2} have been measured during the awake and hibernating phases in about 20 species of mammals with electrodes thermostated to the body temperature of the animal. The results show a constant pH close to 7.4 and a constant Pa_{CO_2} close to 38–60 mmHg. This of course is strikingly different from measurements obtained from poikilotherms over a similar temperature span. The values of pH in this last group are much higher (relative alkalosis) and Pa_{CO_2} much lower than control values obtained in warmer temperatures. The response of hibernators is different because it requires accumulation of CO_2 in order to reduce pH. The response is not peculiar to the buffer choice of the blood in hibernators since it has been shown that the alpha-stat strategy, namely, hyperventilation and relative alkalosis, is adopted in special cases by hibernators when the process of body cooling is not part of hibernation induction, for instance, during the day-to-night cycling in summer. The hibernator's pH and Pa_{CO_2} during the hibernation period cannot be reached from the normothermic state by the sole effect of temperature, such as is the case for the poikilotherms.

In all cases, hibernation is characterized by respiratory acidosis, with a decrease in pH ranging from 0.24 to 0.48 units and a two- to fourfold increase in P_{CO_2} corresponding to accumulation of CO_2 in the blood. The buildup of the respiratory acidosis during entrance into hibernation requires relative hypoventilation. The opposite is observed for the arousal phase. Intracellular determinations of pH have been conducted in different organs of hibernating European hamsters [44]: there, the acidotic load appears to be well distributed by the blood in all extracellular compartments of hibernators, especially the brain and muscle tissues, which constitute by far the largest mass of the body. By contrast, the liver exhibits a different response, and to some extent also the heart, with partial intracellular metabolic compensation that attempts to buffer the pH toward electroneutrality. This difference is significant, since it demonstrates that both mechanisms of pH-stat (brain and muscle) and alpha-stat (liver and heart) may coexist within the same species. This concept demonstrates that, even for the extended range of hypothermic temperatures observed in hibernation, the defenses vary more in a quantitative fashion, rather than in a strict qualitative way. The remarkable feature of this phenomenon, however, lies in the extremely low body temperature reached and the long time for which it is well tolerated.

ACIDOSIS-MEDIATED INHIBITION

It has been suggested [40] that the prevalent respiratory acidosis of hibernation could inhibit both metabolic activity and thermoregulatory mechanisms. If CO_2 is in fact the potential mediator of this inhibition, it enjoys many advantages: it is in fact endogenously created, and it rapidly equilibrates throughout the tissues during accumulation and removal from the body. Specific enzymatic activities, like phosphofructokinase, are inhibited by the maintenance of pH at constant values during the period of temperature reduction. This has been shown to be the main mechanism of energy saving in muscle during hibernation, while the inhibition is less active for the same enzyme in the liver, where intracellular alpha-stat regulation keeps the pH at a higher level [45]. The traditional interpretation of the different regulation in the liver has been that this organ needs to preserve enzymatic functions at a much higher level than muscle, to continue to provide substrates to the body during hibernation. A similar interpretation can apply to the heart, since continuing function of this organ is required, which would be better maintained by alpha-stat rather than by pH-stat strategy. These considerations are pertinent when we envision how they may apply to an adult human during cardiopulmonary bypass.

In the most frequent clinical situation, where hyperthermia is usually rapidly induced after initiation of bypass and when spontaneous beating of cardiac ventricles is not necessary to maintain circulation, but may only contribute to deleterious accumulation of an acid debt, spontaneous utilization of substrates must be rapidly blocked with global myocardial arrest obtained by rapid infusion of cold cardioplegia.

A reversible inhibition of several nervous processes by CO_2 accumulation has also been reported [44, 46]. Conversely, during the arousal phase, the hyperventilation that precedes the maximal temperature rise will rapidly reduce P_{CO_2}, returning tissue pH values toward the traditional alpha-stat situation. This strategy apparently is essential to reach and sustain the very low temperature levels with the maintained ability to reverse this status rapidly. The profound inhibition of metabolic and nervous functions of hibernators appears to offer protection and preservation of organs rather than continuing functional integrity. This property has evolved more recently among mammals and may constitute a valid analogy for correction of pH during cardiac operations in humans.

In addition to the presumptive organ preservation properties of maintaining a constant pH at low temperature, the addition of CO_2 to the oxygenator gases during hypothermic cardiopulmonary bypass has substantial effects on cerebral perfusion.

CEREBRAL FLOW STUDIES

In this area, some human evidence has been collected that can be usefully summarized. Autoregulation of cerebral blood flow (CBF) during cardiopulmonary bypass has been studied during different combinations of pump prime composition, flow regimens, and body temperatures. Henriksen et al. [47] reported that CBF increased during hypothermic bypass, from a prebypass period of 20, up to 66 ml/100 g/min. They attributed such high values of circulatory flow to microembolism with reactive hyperemia. These values differ substantially from the results reported by Govier et al. [48], who during cold cardiopulmonary bypass observed a decrease of 55% in CBF from previous normothermic control levels. Both anesthetic management and acid–base strategy differed widely in these two studies. Henriksen et al. utilized mainly inhalational anesthesia with enflurane for prebypass anesthetic, and *corrected* blood gas values for body temperature, maintaining $Paco_2$ values ranging from 48 to 100 mmHg when measured at 37°C. Govier et al., on the other hand, used a narcotic-based anesthetic and managed arterial blood gases using *uncorrected* values for Pco_2; their values were 35–60 mmHg when measured at 37°C. The data, therefore, may be interpreted as a demonstration that the hypercapnic regimen of the study by Henriksen et al. could have induced a large increase in CBF.

Final verification of such interpretation still needs studies involving large numbers of patients. Meanwhile, in 1985, Roy and Prough [49] directly measured CBF with the radioisotope technique of ^{133}Xe injection into the arterial line of the oxygenator, during cold cardiopulmonary bypass. Their patients were assigned to two contrasting strategies regarding correction of ABG values for temperature. One group of patients was maintained at a $Paco_2$ level close to 40 mmHg when measured at 37°C (uncorrected group) while the other had $Paco_2$ values around 35°C when corrected for temperature (corrected group; the temperature, however, was only lowered to 28.7°C in both groups). The results show that CBF was substantially higher during cold cardiopulmonary bypass for higher $Paco_2$ levels (i.e., the temperature-corrected group, or the group maintained with a pH-stat-type regulation). The uncorrected group (alpha-stat-type regulation) had lower CBFs, all other study variables being closely controlled (perfusion pressure, pump flow, and hematocrit). Despite the clear differences, the principle suggested by these data is not irrefutable, because of the use of moderate hypothermia, with relatively small infringement upon acid–base regulation. The same authors [50] verified this result in another small group of patients during cold cardiopulmonary bypass with even tighter control of CO_2 values (27 or 40 mmHg: equivalent to 40 or 65 mmHg uncorrected for temperature). Both patients groups had CBF measured during controlled reduction of mean pressure from 70 to 50 mmHg following vasodilation with nitroprusside. The group with corrected CO_2 values demonstrated a larger fall in CBF than did the group with uncorrected values. The authors postulate a loss of autoregulation in the group with corrected CO_2 (higher CO_2 levels) though they warn in their discussion that these data should not indicate that correction of ABG may lead to cerebral ischemia. Similarly, Rogers et al. [51] showed that phenylephrine infusion increased significantly mean arterial pressures and CBF in patients who were managed during cold cardiopulmonary bypass at corrected $Paco_2$ levels. While these data support the hypothesis that autoregulation is lost when CO_2 temperature correction is used during moderate $(26°-27°C)$ hypothermia, it is obvious that CBF is much larger, usually by a factor of 2, in all groups of patients in which $Paco_2$ is elevated (or a strategy of pH-stat, or temperature correction, is pursued), compared with the noncorrected groups. Similar considerations apply to the study by Murkin et al. [29], who assessed CBF in association with direct determination of cerebral oxygen consumption in patients studied at different times during hypothermic cardiopulmonary bypass. This last study included two large groups of patients maintained at different $Paco_2$ regimens, corrected for temperature (with addition of CO_2 to the oxygenator gas) or uncorrected. In this study, no significant difference is demonstrated in cerebral oxygen consumption between the two groups at any time of study, not even during the hypothermic phase of extracorporeal circulation, although $CMRo_2$ was significantly reduced in both groups during hypothermia. Blood flow in the "corrected group" (high CO_2) remained 2–3 times higher than in the group maintained at low CO_2. In the discussion, the authors comment that "the maintenance of a temperature corrected $Paco_2$ of 40 mmHg (pH-stat) during hypothermic by-pass uncouples the relationship between CBF and $CMRo_2$ and produces a pressure-passive CBF system. Maintaining a temperature uncorrected $Paco_2$ of 40 mmHg (alpha-stat) preserves cerebral autoregulation allowing CBF to be determined by $CMRo_2$, independent of perfusion pressure over the range of 20 to 100 mmHg."

The arguments from the cerebral flow studies that higher (corrected) $Paco_2$ levels go hand in hand with a loss of autoregulation in our opinion ignore that high $Paco_2$ levels are usually accompanied by much higher CBFs and appear safer than noncorrecting regimens, particularly if hemodilution if used.

CONCLUSION

Unquestionably, correction of Po_2 for body temperature is most appropriate. Lack of correction may lead to serious overestimation of arterial and especially venous Po_2. Because of changes in blood flow distribution, an increase in diffusion distance for Po_2 may occur. Therefore it is extremely important to maintain high Pao_2 and $P\bar{v}o_2$. Use of uncorrected values, which are artifactually high during hypothermia, may thus result in a false sense of security.

Regarding pH correction, the decision to correct or not correct pH for temperature cannot be based only on the available evidence suggesting that physiological and enzymatic *function* is better maintained with noncorrection. The other important issue is organ *preservation* during the sojourn at low temperature. As pointed out by Hochachka [52], many similarities exist between the biological characteristics of tolerance to hypoxia and tolerance to hypothermia. Preservation of membrane integrity and active regulation of metabolism during hypothermia are both requirements of any strategy of cellular protection during hypothermia. The effects of pH on most of the components of these functions are as yet unknown. What is known is that cerebral blood flow is higher during hypothermia with correction. Furthermore, hibernating mammals use a correcting strategy for those organs that require preservation rather than function during hypothermia (e.g., brain and muscle).

Therefore, based on currently available knowledge, when *preservation* is important, rather than function (e.g., during the stable period of cardiopulmonary bypass when the aorta is cross-clamped), correction of pH is most appropriate. Uncorrected pH should not be used until *function* again becomes more important, at the end of the bypass period when optimal cardiac output is required. Alternatively, when special techniques are used, such as surface cooling in infants before the stable bypass period, when spontaneous contractility and avoidance of arrhythmias are crucial to tissue perfusion, a noncorrection plan is superior. This, however, can only be applied over a relatively small temperature range. A definitive answer to the question must await the investigation of pH on various metabolic and membrane-stabilizing cellular functions. The overall effects of various pH values on the overall morbidity of hypothermic cardiopulmonary bypass will probably not be assessable until further data are available.

REFERENCES

1. Severinghaus JW, Larson CP Jr: Respiration in anesthesia. In: Fenn WO, Rahn H (eds) Handbook of physiology, vol 2. Sect 3: Respiration. American Physiological Society, Washington DC, 1965, pp 1219–1264.
2. Rahn H, Reeves RB, Howell BJ: Hydrogen ion regulation, temperature, and evolution. Am Rev Respir Dis 112:165–172, 1975.
3. Reeves RB, Rahn H: Patterns in vertebrate acid–base regulation. In: Wood SC, Lenfant C (eds) Evolution and respiratory processes: a comparative approach. Marcel Dekker, New York, 1979, pp 225–252.

4. Goodrich CA: Acid–base balance in ectothermic and hibernating marmots. Am J Physiol 224:1185, 1973.
5. Merrill EW, Gilliland ER, Cokelet G, et al.: Rheology of human blood, near and at zero flow: effects of temperature and hematocrit level. Biophys J 3:199–213, 1963.
6. Steen PA, Soule EH, Michenfelder JD: Detrimental effect of prolonged hypothermia in cats and monkeys with and without regional cerebral ischemia. Stroke 10:522–529, 1979.
7. Gorden RJ, Ravin M, Daicoff GR, et al.: Effects of hemodilution on hypotension during cardiopulmonary bypass. Anesth Analg 54:482–488, 1975.
8. Siesjo BK: Brain energy metabolism. Wiley, New York, 1978, pp 446–449.
9. Thomas EJ, Marshall J, Ross-Russell RW, et al.: Effect of hematocrit on cerebral blood-flow in man. Lancet 2:941–943, 1977.
10. Lafferty JJ, Keykhah MM, Shapiro HM, et al.: Cerebral hypometabolism obtained with deep pentobarbital anesthesia and hypothermia (30°C). Anesthesiology 49:159–164, 1978.
11. Steen PA, Michenfelder JD: Barbiturate protection in tolerant and nontolerant hypoxic mice: comparison with hypothermic protection. Anesthesiology 50:404–408, 1979.
12. White RJ: Cerebral hypothermia and circulatory arrest: review and commentary, Mayo Clin Proc 53:450–458, 1978.
13. White FN: A comparative physiological approach to hypothermia. J Thorac Cardiovasc Surg 82:821–831, 1981.
14. Banchik ME, Blancato LS: Correlation of esophageal, rectal and pulmonary artery temperature measurement during rapid extracorporeal cooling. Anesthesiology [Suppl 3A] 65:A531, 1986.
15. Harris EA, Seelye ER, Squire AW: Oxygen consumption during cardiopulmonary bypass with moderate hypothermia in man. Br J Anaesth 43:1113–1120, 1971.
16. Noback CR, Tinker JH: Hypothermia after cardiopulmonary bypass in man. Anesthesiology 53:277–280, 1980.
17. Niemenen MT, Rosow CE, Triantafillow A, et al.: Temperature gradients in cardiac surgical patients: a comparison of halothane and fentanyl. Anesth Analg 62:1002–1005, 1983.
18. Ross BA, Lord Brock, Aynsley-Green A: Observations on central and peripheral temperatures in the understanding and management of shock. Br J Surg 56:877–882, 1969.
19. Sladen RN: Temperature and ventilation after hypothermic cardiopulmonary bypass. Anesth Analg 64:816–820, 1985.
20. Christoforides C, Hedley-Whyte J: Effect of temperature and hemoglobin concentration on solubility of O_2 in blood. J Appl Physiol 27:592–596, 1969.
21. Hlastala MP, Woodson RD, Wranne B: Influence of temperature on hemoglobin–ligand interaction in whole blood. J Appl Physiol 43:545–550, 1977.
22. Nunn JF, Bergman NA, Bunatyan A, Coleman AJ: Temperature coefficients for Pco_2 and Po_2 of blood in vitro. J Appl Physiol 20:23–26, 1965.
23. Severinghaus JW: Blood gas calculator. J Appl Physiol 21:1108–1116, 1966.
24. Thomas LT Jr: Algorithms for selected blood acid–base and blood gas calculations. J Appl Physiol 33:154–158, 1972.
25. Severinghaus JW, Stafford M, Thunstrom AM: Estimation of skin metabolism and blood flow with $TcPo_2$ and $TcPco_2$ electrodes by cuff occlusion of the circulation. Acta Anaesth Scand [Suppl] 68:9–15, 1978.
26. National Committee for Clinical Laboratory Standards: Tentative standard for definitions of quantities and conventions related to blood pH and gas analysis. NCCLS pub 2:329–361, 1982.
27. Spurr GB, Hutt BK, Horvath SM: Responses of dogs to hypothermia. Am J Physiol 179:139–145, 1954.
28. Rosomoff HL, Holaday DA: Cerebral blood flow and cerebral oxygen comsumption during hypothermia. Am J Physiol 179:85–88, 1954.
29. Murkin JM, Farrar JK, Tweed WA, et al.: Acid–base management during hypothermic cardiopulmonary bypass profoundly influences cerebral blood flow and cerebral autoregulation. Anesthesiology [Suppl 3A] 65:A320, 1986.
30. Tenney SM: A theoretical analysis of the relationship between venous blood and mean tissue oxygen pressures. Respir Physiol 20:283–296, 1974.
31. Adolf EF: Effects of low body temperature on tissue oxygen utilization. In: Dripps RD (ed) The physiology of induced hypothermia. National Academy of Sciences–National Research

Council, Washington DC, 1956, pp 44–49.

32. Jöbsis FF, Noninvasive, infrared monitoring of cerebral and myocardial oxygen sufficiency and circulatory parameters. Science 198:1264–1267, 1977.
33. Reeves RB: What are normal acid–base conditions in man when body temperature changes? In: Rahn H, Parkash O (eds) Acid base regulation and body temperature. Martinus Nijhoff, Boston, 1985, pp 13–32.
34. Reeves RB: Temperature–induced changes in blood acid–base status: pH and Pco_2 in a binary buffer. J Appl Physiol 40:752–761, 1976.
35. Howell BJ, Baumgardner F, Bondi K, Rahn H: Acid–base balance in cold-blooded vertebrates as a function of body temperature. Am J Physiol 218:600–606, 1970.
36. Reeves RB: Temperature-induced changes in blood acid–base status: Donnan r_{cl} and red cell volume. J Appl Physiol 40:762–767, 1976.
37. Poole-Wilson PA, Langer GA: Effects of acidosis on mechanical function and Ca^{2+} exchange in rabbit myocardium. Am J Physiol 236:H525–H533, 1979.
38. Swain JA, White FN, Peters RM: The effect of pH on the hypothermic fibrillation threshold. J Thor and Cardio Surgery, 87:445–451, 1984.
39. Buckberg GD, Brazier JR, Nelson RL, et al.: Studies of the effects of hypothermia on regional myocardial blood flow and metabolism during cardiopulmonary bypass. I. The adequately perfused beating, fibrillating and arrested heart. J Thorac Cardiovasc Surg 73:87–94, 1977.
40. Buckberg GD, Becker H, Vinten-Johansen, J, et al.: Myocardial function resulting from varying acid–base management during and following deep surface and perfusion hypothermia and circulatory arrest. In: Rahn H, Prakash O (eds) Acid base regulation and body temperature. Martinus Nijhoff, Boston, 1985, pp 135–159.
41. Malan A: Acid–base regulation during hibernation. In: Rahn H, Prakash O (eds) Acid–base regulation and body temperature. Martinus Nijhoff, Boston, 1985, pp 33–53.
42. Malan A: Enzyme regulation, metabolic rate and acid–base state in hibernation. In: Gilles R (ed) Animals and environmental fitness. Pergamon, Oxford, 1980, pp 487–501.
43. Kayser C, Malan A: Central nervous system and hibernation. Experientia 19:1–11, 1963.
44. Malan A, Rodeau JL, Doull R: Intracellular pH in hibernating hamsters. Cryobiology 18: 100–101, 1981.
45. Hand SC, Somero GN: Phosphofructokinase of the hibernator *Citellus beecheyi*: temperature and pH regulation of activity via influences on the tetramer–dimer equilibrium. Physiol Zool 56:380–388, 1983.
46. Kilduff TS, Sharp FR, Heller HC: ^{14}C 2-deoxyglucose uptake in ground squirrel brain during hibernation. J Neurosci 2:143–157, 1982.
47. Henriksen L, Hjelms E, Lindeburgh T: Brain perfusion during cardiac operations. J Thorac Cardiovasc Surg 86:202–208, 1983.
48. Govier AV, Reves JG, McKay RD, et al.: Factors and their influence on regional cerebral blood flow during nonpulsatile cardiopulmonary bypass. Ann Thorac Surg 38:592–600, 1984.
49. Roy RC, Prough DS, Stump DA, Williams T, Gravlee GP, Mills SA, Howard G: Cerebral blood flow response to CO_2 during extracorporeal circulation under high-dose fentanyl anesthesia. Anesthesiology [Suppl 3A] 63:A43, 1985.
50. Prough DS, Stump DA, Rogers AT, Gravlee GP, Angert KC: Nitroprusside decreases cerebral blood flow during cardiopulmonary bypass. Anesthesiology [Suppl 3A] 65:A13, 1986.
51. Rogers AT, Gravlee GP, Prough DS, Stump DA, Augert KC: Cerebral autoregulation is impaired during cardiopulmonary bypass. Anesthesiology [Suppl 3A] 65:A12, 1986.
52. Hochachka PW: Defense strategies against hypoxia and hypothermia. Science 231:234–241, 1986.

4. BLOOD GASES SHOULD NOT BE TEMPERATURE CORRECTED DURING HYPOTHERMIA

PAUL L. GOLDINER
YASU OKA
EDWARD SVADJIAN

A discussion of acid–base balance usually concerns the hydrogen ion regulation of the extracellular environment, i.e., the blood or hemolymph that bathes the cells. Usually we accept a pH of 7.40 and a Pco_2 of 40 mmHg values as somehow "determined by nature," assuming that, as long as such data are preserved, the intracellular hydrogen ion concentration is appropriately regulated. Back in 1958, Bernard Davis [1] stated that the ideal status for the intermediary metabolism of cells is the state of neutrality. He surveyed the ionization constants of several hundred water-soluble biosynthetic intermediates and found with few exceptions that the dissociation constant (pK) for the acid compounds was less than 4.60 and for the basic compounds more than 9.20.

These intermediary compounds are completely ionized in the region around neutrality and have little tendency to escape from the cell across the plasma membrane. On the other hand, a few metabolites, uncharged at neutrality, are found only as excretory or fermentation products. Davis proved that complete ionization is an efficient retention mechanism for metabolites within the cell or organelle. This is elegantly expressed by the title of his paper, "On the importance of being ionized."

Recently it has been recognized that stability of acid–base balance is achieved not just through the constancy of blood pH, but by the preservation of protein net charge states in extracellular and intracellular compartments. Regulation of acid–base balance as temperature varies can now be related to the preservation of cellular activities dependent on protein function, because the binding of different substrates, activators, and inhibitors to protein enzyme and transport molecules is directly affected by charge distribution. Furthermore, Donnan equilibria, which are key factors in ion and water distribution, also depend on protein net charge states.

These considerations suggest that the constancy of the internal environment as now perceived did not suddenly emerge with the achievement of homeothermism; rather the *milieu interieur* of Claude Bernard has been carefully regulated throughout vertebrate development so as to preserve body protein activities. The pH change resulting from the temperature-altered dissociation strength of histidine imidazole groups affects the carbonic acid bicarbonate equilibrium, together with the effect of temperature on carbon dioxide solubility. These simultaneous changes can be described and quantitatively predicted from simple chemical equilibrium and mass conservation equations [2, 3]. Proteins contain only one additional ionizing group titratable in the physiological pH range, the N-terminal alpha-amino group, in addition to the histidine imidazolium group. However, the small number of alpha-amino groups compared to histidine imidazole groups, combined with a similar large range of ionization, permits all proteins for simplified purposes to be treated as though only histidine imidazole is making a contribution when pH varies in the physiological range. Thus, if alpha-imidazole can be computed for the conditions occurring for blood in a syringe, a measure of the change in mean net protein charge can be obtained.

INTRACELLULAR pH

As it was stated above, neutrality or near neutrality is the intracellular state that must be regulated and defended in order to maintain complete ionization of low molecular weight, water-soluble biosynthetic intermediates to provide a mechanism for their maximal retention within the cell membrane. This neutrality is achieved by the regulation of the external environment that bathes the cell and tissue. It is well known that the dissociation of water is profoundly affected by temperature. The pH of neutrality, or 0.5 pKw (dissociation constant for water), is nearly 7.50 at 0°C and 6.80 at 37°C. If intracellular neutrality is indeed to be maintained at various body temperatures, then the intracellular pH should shift proportionally [4]. Reeves and Wilson [5] and Malan et al. [6] studied the range of 48 intracellular pH values of skeletal muscle for two ectotherms acclimatized at temperatures between 5°C and 31°C. This study also includes the literature values for muscle pH of man, dog, and rat ($n = 184$) at 37°C, which shows that the pH increases with body cooling and follows closely change in neutrality of water. These observations tend to support the hypothesis of Davis [1], but they also require an intracellular buffer mechanism that will not only attach the intracellular pH to the region of neutrality, but will also change its pK with temperature parallel to the changes in neutrality of water.

Responsible for this behavior is the protein buffering, largely imidazole, of histidine acting together with the bicarbonate and phosphate buffering. Summarizing the literature data, it can be stated that the intracellular pH changes but remains neutral, and the net charge of the dissociation of the imidazole buffer remains constant. It is also important to point out that, in spite of the large changes that Pco_2 undergoes with temperature, the CO_2 content of the muscles in the ectotherm remains essentially constant [7, 8]. Therefore, we are not confronted with loading and unloading of CO_2 stores as the body warms or cools, but only with changes in pH and Pco_2.

EXTRACELLULAR pH

Behavior of human blood

For human blood treated as though it were a single-phase binary buffer, an approximation that permits prediction of changes of pH and Pco_2 in this system as temperature varies, the calculated variation of alpha-imidazole over the temperature range $0°-45°C$ is almost negligible [9]. In this system, protein net charge is essentially invariant as temperature changes at constant CO_2 content. Reeves and Malan [9] experimentally tested this conclusion by measuring the *Donnan distribution* between human red blood cells and plasma for Cl^- under in vitro conditions; even though pH changed from 7.30 to 7.95 as temperature changed, chloride ion distribution between red blood cells and plasma water remained constant. This experiment established that the protein CO_2-bicarbonate binary buffer mixture of plasma and whole blood has the remarkable property at constant CO_2 content of maintaining a protein charge state invariant when temperature changes, even though pH and Pco_2 vary significantly. Thus these computations establish that, in the open metabolizing system, alpha-imidazole is regulated by the animal so as to maintain constant protein charge state. To be able to compare this system of acid–base regulation with the constant pH system of homeotherms, the ectotherm pattern of acid–base control has been termed *alphastat regulation* [7]. This suggests that, by whatever means the intact animal regulates his acid–base balance as body temperature changes, alpha-imidazole, and thus mean protein net charge, are protected and maintained constant.

If cells are to defend their neutrality and also to eliminate their acid metabolites and CO_2, they must be provided with a circulating environment that is relatively more alkaline. At $37°C$, the intracellular H^+ concentration at neutrality is 160 nM/L (pH 6.80) and that of blood 40 nM/L (pH 7.40). Thus, between cells and blood, man maintains a considerable H^+ gradient. The behavior of blood in vitro was reported by Rahn [10], who presented values of some 35 species of vertebrates acclimated at various temperatures, including the normothermic birds, mammals, and man.

It has been shown that the blood band runs parallel to that of the muscle tissue and thus the mean Δ pH is about 0.7 units, which is equivalent to an intracellular pH–extracellular pH ratio of 5:1. We, therefore, see that blood is regulated to maintain what has been called a constant relative alkalinity that is relative to the neutrality of water [11]. This relationship can also be expressed numerically by saying that the ratio of OH^- to H^+ in the blood is about 20:1, which is calculated by obtaining the antilog of 2 (pH blood − pH neutrality). Thus, we see that the regulation of blood pH in ectotherms appears to be regulated in such a way that at all temperatures it is more alkaline than the intracellular pH, and that the pH between cells and blood remains constant. Peters and Van Slyke [12] expressed this fact five decades earlier in the following way: for "a state compatible with life the reaction of the inner fluids must be slightly to the alkaline side of the neutral point."

Our skin is normally at a temperature of about 33°C and on a cold day our exposed skin can actually be quite comfortable at 20°C or below. Our liver normally operates 1°C above core temperature and during exercise our deep muscle temperature will reach values of 41°C. Thus, on a cold and windy day, an exercising person may exhibit local temperatures that may differ by as much as 20°C or more. The normal arterial blood will leave at a core temperature of 37°C, but will cool or warm to the specific temperatures of the peripheral tissues before exchange at the capillary level occurs. During this transition, the blood behaves in the same way as it would had it been cooled or warmed in vitro.

Blood in vitro

Blood enclosed in vitro in the absence of gas exchange must necessarily have a constant carbon dioxide content. Does blood, or more accurately, true plasma, in vivo have a constant CO_2 content? Since most (98%) of the carbon dioxide in true plasma is in the chemical form of bicarbonate ions, one can ask the equivalent question: are plasma bicarbonate concentrations unchanged as air-breathing ectotherms change body temperature?

Robin [13] found an increase in bicarbonate concentration as body temperature rose in the turtle. Howell et al. [11] reported that bicarbonate concentrations fell as body temperature rose in poikilotherms. In both cases, the bicarbonate concentrations were calculated by the Henderson–Hasselbach equation from measured pH and PCO_2 data. In experiments in which total carbon dioxide content was measured directly by Van Slyke analysis [12], plasma CO_2 content did not change significantly as body temperature was altered. Thus, in air-breathing ectotherms, neither loading nor unloading of blood carbon dioxide stores takes place during alteration of body temperature [7].

It is well known from the empirical observations reported by Rosenthal [14] that blood removed at 37°C and cooled in vitro will increase its pH. Reeves [3] has reinvestigated the behavior of blood as it is warmed and cooled in order to record not only the pH and PCO_2, but also to determine whether a change occurs in the Donnan ratio; this is because at 37°C any change in pH will have a profound effect upon the redistribution of electrolytes between cell and plasma, accounting also for changes in red cell volume. He was able to demonstrate that, although pH and P_{CO_2} undergo marked changes, the Cl^- distribution between cells and plasma remains unaltered and, therefore, the HCO_3^- distribution remains unaltered as well. It is therefore not surprising that no change in red cell volume occurs. Thus, cells and plasma appear to behave independently; whereas the H^+ concentration is diminished with cooling, the OH^- concentration and relative alkalinity are preserved. The CO_2 tension decreases not only because of the increase in solubility and the change in pK of the HCO_3^- buffer system, but also because of the increase in pH [15].

To explain these reactions, we can no longer take refuge in the bicarbonate buffer system, but must turn our attention to its simultaneous interaction with the protein buffer. Reeves [16] has shown the dominant effect of the protein buffers. Of all the protein-dissociable groups that are available, it is only imidazole of histidine and a small contribution of N-terminal alpha-amino groups that have the proper pK and whose pK changes to the same degree with temperature as the observed changes in blood neutrality.

The hypothermic or hyperthermic behavior of blood in normal man

In vitro analysis of acid–base balance as blood changes temperature suggests that characterization of the pH dependence on temperature in vivo as a linear function may be inappropriate. If acid–base regulation in vivo is based on regulation of alpha-imidazole, description of the nonlinear dependence of blood pH on temperature by use of a single $\Delta pH/\Delta t°$ will neither describe the regulation observed nor assist in comparing one system with another.

As indicated above, the blood that leaves the core at 37°C will either cool or warm on its way to our peripheral tissues. Before it arrives at the precapillary level, it will therefore behave as blood in vitro [15]. The skin blood has a pH of 7.60 and a P_{CO_2} of 22 mmHg, whereas the exercising muscle operates at a blood pH of 7.35 and a P_{CO_2} of 48 mmHg. In spite of these changes, the CO_2 and HCO_3^- content, the net charge of the imidazole buffer, the Donnan ratio, and the relative alkalinity or OH^-/H^+ ratio are unaltered. We can assume that at least in the skin the ratio of intracellular hydrogen ion to extracellular hydrogen ion is also normal and the intracellular pH is close to neutrality at 25°C. According to this concept, it is difficult to explain these local conditions in terms of alkalosis or acidosis if indeed the primary goals are to maintain a neutral pH within the tissues and have them perfused by a fluid that is slightly to the alkaline side.

Constant relative alkalinity

Rahn [17] pointed out that at first analysis it hardly appears that acid–base balance regulation occurs in ectotherms because of the dependence of pH and P_{CO_2} on body temperature. He noted, however, that they were the defended parameters. Water is by definition neutral when $(OH^-) = (H^+)$, or $(OH^-):$ $(H^+) = 1$ or pH = pOH. Since pH + pOH = pKw at neutrality (pN), 2 pN = pKw or pN = $\frac{1}{2}$ pKw. The dissociation of water expressed by pKw is a function of temperature ranging from 14.94 at 0°C to 13.53 at 40°C; thus pN is also temperature dependent, with neutrality being 7.47 at 0°C and 6.77 at 40°C. Extracelluar fluids, including blood, are alkaline solutions, blood pH and pN. Howell [11] and Rahn et al. [4] documented the parallel between blood pH and pN as body temperature changes; under these conditions, blood pH = pN + K where the constant K is about 0.6–0.8 units. When blood pH–pN remains constant, the OH^-:H^+ ratio, or relative alkalinity, is also constant.

Just as in alphastat control (ectothermic animals), constant relative alkalinity would have to be actively regulated by physiological processes, and Pco_2 control in air-breathing vertebrates would necessarily be the means of effecting a constant relative alkalinity.

Ventilatory control of abid–base balance

Previous summaries of blood values have shown that open regulated systems in vivo and closed systems in vitro (at constant CO_2 content) have essentially identical pH and Pco_2 variation with temperature. In the open system, with the metabolizing animal continuously producing carbon dioxide, the pattern of acid–base regulation requires that the animal's ventilation be adjusted at each temperature to provide the proper Pco_2. Looking at the alveolar equation $\dfrac{\dot{V}a}{\dot{V}co_2} = K\,\dfrac{1}{Pco_2}$ where $\dot{V}a$ is alveolar ventilation, $\dot{V}co_2$ carbon dioxide production, and K is a constant, it is evident that, for carbon dioxide tension to decrease as body temperature falls, it is necessary for the ratio $\dot{V}a$:$\dot{V}co_2$ to increase; that is, the ventilation per unit of metabolism, or relative ventilation, must increase as temperature falls [10].

Experimental data in accord with this analysis have been provided by Jackson [18]. At a body temperature of 10°C, blood CO_2 tension had decreased to 14 mmHg, while relative ventilation, $\dot{V}_E$:$\dot{V}o_2$ had doubled. Hence, the ventilation per unit oxygen consumption increased as body temperature fell, essentially hyperventilating as temperature decreased. The most remarkable observation in these experiments was that $\dot{V}_E$ was essentially constant over the 20°C range; the value of the ratio $\dot{V}_E$:$\dot{V}o_2$ changed due to changes in oxygen consumption. By adding carbon dioxide to the inspired air, Jackson et al. [19], in turtles, and Davies and Kopetzky [20], in alligators, were able to establish $\dot{V}_E$ sensitivity to $Paco_2$ at several body temperatures; increased $Paco_2$ produced a marked hyperventilation at all temperatures. Jackson and Silverblatt [21] followed the response of turtles to long-lasting (2–4 h) experimental dives at constant body temperature (24°C). Immediately after the dive, a brisk hyperventilation restored blood pH to normal in 2 h despite a continuing metabolic acidosis. These experiments indicate the power of ventilatory control of blood carbon dioxide tensions to maintain a normal blood pH setpoint both when temperature is the experimental variable and when a metabolic acidosis from a prolonged apnea challenges the regulated acid–base balance.

Temperature-sensitive ventilation receptor

How is ventilation regulated in these circumstances? What is the receptor that controls ventilation and establishes the correct $\dot{V}_E$ for the challenge imposed, i.e., temperature change or isothermal metabolic acidosis?

Reeves [7] suggested that both types of regulation could be achieved if the ventilation receptor had two fundamental properties: (a) the receptor must contain a dissociable group with a pK in the physiological range conferring pH responsiveness, and (b) the change in pK with temperature for that group must be similar to the in vivo blood pH temperature curve, i.e., a $\Delta H°$ of 7 kcal/mol [22]. It is then possible to look at the receptor site as a specific amino acid in a protein component whose charge state and conformation are sensitive to the animal's acid–base status at any body temperature. The protein might be considered as an *ion-gating protein* in the membrane of a respiratory pacemaker neuron; the dissociation of the receptor site is accepted in terms of a histidine imidazole group in peptide linkage, unique among biological compounds for satisfying the two important conditions already mentioned.

Intracellular pH responses to changing body temperature

If the central function of ectotherm acid–base balance is protection of protein charge states, and thus protein activity, as body temperature varies, how does extracellular acid–base regulation affect the bulk of protein function in the organism, i.e., intracellular proteins?

In their experimental study done in 1976, Malan et al. [23] indicate that, even though intracellular pH values are not equilibrium distributions for H^+ (and/or HCO_3^- and OH^-) but are actively maintained near neutrality, the change in pH with changing body temperature follows the path of near-constant alpha-imidazole. These findings emphasize that the observed pattern of regulation of CO_2 partial pressure when body temperature changes not only regulates and preserves peptide histidine imidazole dissociation in the extracellular compartment, but also within cells as well.

Hence, Donnan states and protein activities are shielded from, rather than disrupted by, temperature fluctuations.

Wood and Moberly [24] studied the influence of temperature on the respiratory properties of the lizard to express the acid–base responses to a 30°C body temperature change. The 30°C rise of body temperature is associated with a change in blood pH from 7.93 (5°C) to 7.47 (33°C); despite these dramatic changes in blood pH, protein histidine dissociation and relative alkalinity remain constant. The corresponding change in partial pressure of CO_2 is 5.8–23.7 Torr; when temperature and carbon dioxide partial pressure change simultaneously under these conditions, no titration of protein buffers forming additional bicarbonate occurs. These acid–base changes can be accomplished quickly and reversibly because they require no extensive loading or unloading of carbon dioxide either from tissue or blood stores.

Dramatic changes in body temperature can be accommodated with essentially no change in blood or intracellular protein net charge state. The special properties of CO_2–HCO_3^- and protein binary buffer systems well as the regulation of ventilation permit the animal the freedom to change body temperature rapidly and not suffer transients to alpha-imidazole in either direction. It is this protection from large changes in net charge of cellular proteins that, in part at least, permits the lizard, in Barcroft's words, to "so control its reactions as to keep them in step over a great range of temperature."

Ectothermic vertebrates exhibit a *fixité du milieu interieur* no less striking than the functionally related regulation of blood pH by mammalian and avian species. When the factors affecting protein charge state, the dissociation of protein imidazole groups (alpha-imidazole), were examined, it was found that each uniquely defended blood pH at different body temperatures, which is precisely what is required to maintain constant protein charge states.

The implications of a strategy of defending protein charge state in an organism whose biochemical apparatus is composed of protein components, the functions of which critically depend on charge state, are evident. As a single temperature, i.e., 37°C, defense of protein imidazole charge state, alphastat regulation, cannot be distinguished from regulation of blood pH. Hence, homeotherms are not exceptions to alphastat control; they are isothermal examples of the same phenomenon. The Pco_2 passively generated by temperature change closely matches the Pco_2 that must be provided by ventilatory control when the tissue functions as an open CO_2-producing system. This special property of passively responding to a temperature change in a way that maintains constant protein charge state obviates the need for filling or emptying tissue carbon dioxide stores. The passive tissue-buffering properties permit steady-state acid–base conditions to prevail as rapidly as tissue temperature can be altered.

Before discussing the possible use of the above-mentioned principles for the treatment of a patient undergoing hypothermic cardiopulmonary bypass, it is of interest to review briefly the behavior of ectothermic animals when their body temperature is lowered. Actually it is an open system in which the pH and Pco_2 values depend upon the relative ventilation. Comparing the in vivo pH and Pco_2 changes in such ectotherms [11, 25] with the in vitro behavior of blood in man, a striking parallelism was found. What this tells us is that, at any body temperature and its associated metabolic rate, the ventilation is adjusted in such a way as to preserve a constant relative alkalinity and a constant net charge of the imidazole of histidine buffer. It is this state that keeps CO_2 stores of blood and tissues constant and preserves the Donnan ratio, but it does require a relative increase in ventilation or decrease in Pco_2 as the body temperature decreases.

In the past, many regimens have been used for support of the hypothermic patient in the operating room. Literature, data, and our clinical findings suggest that one would try to maintain a constant CO_2 content of the blood, a normal Donnan ratio between plasma and cells, a tissue pH close to neutrality and, last but not least, a constant net charge of the protein buffer, imidazole of histidine. As it was shown for the in vivo (ectothermic) curves of blood, this can be achieved only by lowering the arterial P_{CO_2} sufficiently so that the blood will retain a constant relative alkalinity. In practice, it means the pulmonary ventilation should probably be maintained at or near the euthermic setting as the body is cooled. Under such conditions, the arterial P_{CO_2} will decrease automatically as the metabolic rate is reduced. To monitor the proper ventilation, one need only withdraw a blood sample, rewarm it immediately, and obtain a pH reading on the temperature-controlled meter at 37°C. This value may then be interpreted in the conventional manner. If such a pH value is the same as the previous normothermic data of the patient before cooling, e.g., 7.40, then the desired ventilation and P_{CO_2} are achieved to maintain a constant relative alkalinity. If such a patient's blood has been withdrawn at a core temperature of 20°C and analyzed at that temperature, the pH would have been 7.65 and the P_{CO_2} 18 mmHg if the relative neutrality had been preserved. However, if that sample had been quickly rewarmed anaerobically and measured at 37°C, the pH would then read 7.40 and the P_{CO_2} 40 mmHg.

EVOLUTION OF OUR BUFFER SYSTEM

Detailed investigation of the literature shows that there is no essential difference in acid–base regulation between ectotherms and endotherms except that they operate the same basic buffer systems at two different temperatures, and, therefore, at a different pH.

In figure 4-1, we see the in vivo behavior of our vertebrate ancestors as a function of body temperature. It must be noted that the change in pH with temperature is approximately the same in all the species, although the absolute pH at a given temperature may differ between species. With change in temperature, the relative alkalinity remains constant, as does the difference between the pH of blood and the pH of neutrality.

Of all combinations of amino acids that nature has contrived, there appears to be only one buffer, imidazole of histidine, whose pK is close to 7.0 and $\Delta H°$ is 7 kcal/mol; this allows its pK to change with temperature to essentially the same degree as the pH changes in neutrality of water (figure 4-2). Imidazole of histidine exists in sufficient concentration in our blood (30 mM per liter in plasma) to dominate the other buffer systems. However, to achieve neutrality within the cells and a constant relative alkalinity within the blood, it has to be supported by proper ventilation or P_{CO_2} at every body temperature. Thus, when homeotherms, and finally man, developed in the course of evolution, the archaic buffer system served them well. At 37°C, the tissue pH remains close to neutrality or 6.80 and, according to our inherited tradition, the extracellular fluid is maintained 0.6–0.8 units higher to provide the relatively alkaline environment of 7.40 and a constant intracellular pH–extracellular pH ratio.

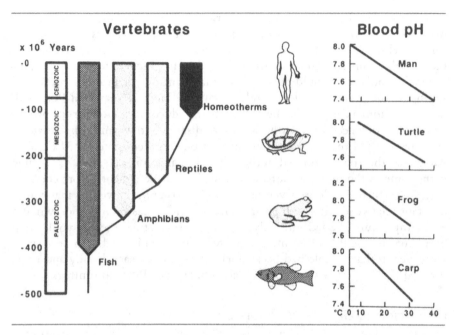

Figure 4-1. For man the in vitro, and for other vertebrates the in vivo, behavior of blood pH as a function of body temperature, suggesting that no basic changes in the blood buffering system have occurred during evolution.

The above-mentioned hydrogen ion regulation is based on the preservation of neutrality of the intracellular state, which is governed by the dissociation of water and is regulated by the compliant protein buffer, imidazole of histidine. The extracellular environment acts as a sink for the acid metabolites of the tissue and is maintained at a constant alkalinity relative to neutrality. The difference between the pH of the extracellular environment and that of neutrality (pN) appears to be constant for a given species and varies between 0.6 to 0.8 pH units. It can be designated aSK. We may describe in a simple way, as shown in figure 4-3, the acid–base regulation of all animals at any body temperature at which the intracellular hydrogen ion concentration is represented by pN and that of the extracellular fluid as pN + K. This relationship is achieved through the interaction of a multibuffer system that not only requires the unique properties of the protein buffer, imidazole of histidine, but also the precise regulation of the bicarbonate buffer ratio by proper ventilation and renal control.

CLINICAL IMPLICATIONS

Clinical use of general body hypothermia in cardiac surgery, which actually originated in the early 1950s, continues to become even more popular today. Modern technology of blood gas measurements assures accurate values of the

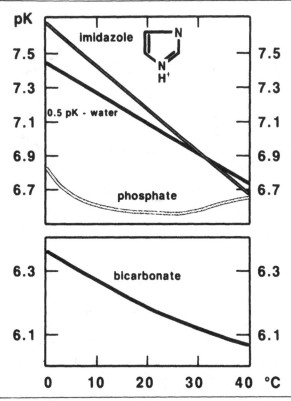

Figure 4-2. Changes in the dissociation constants: pK of CO_2-bicarbonate, phosphate, and imidazole with temperature. The 0.5 pK of water, or neutrality, is also shown.

P_{O_2}, P_{CO_2}, and pH of in vitro samples, providing there is no discrepancy between patient body temperature and the temperature of the blood sample at the time of analysis. During hypothermic cardiopulmonary bypass, the majority of clinical laboratories use arterial and venous blood gas measurements corrected for body temperature. However, controversy exists regarding the necessity to apply temperature correction to blood gas values, originating in part from the hesitancy to add further mathematical complexity to an already difficult subject that could become intimidating to most medical personnel.

It is generally agreed that, at normal body temperature (37°C), ideal values of arterial pH and P_{CO_2} are 7.40 and 40 mmHg, respectively [26]. However, ideal (normal) values for a hypothermic patient are practically unknown. Previous reports describe nomograms [27–31] and computer programs [32] designated to calculate and correct arterial or venous blood gas values and pH for temperature discrepancies.

When a blood specimen with a known pH and P_{CO_2} is cooled anaerobically to a lower temperature, the P_{CO_2} decreases and the pH increases in a

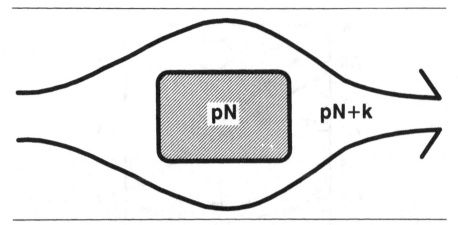

Figure 4-3. A simple description of acid–base regulation in animals and man at any normal body temperature at which pN is the neutrality of the intracellular environment and pN + k is the extracellular enviornment.

predictable manner. This has been formulated by Severinghaus [29, 30] and others and is applied by clinicians to correct the pH and P_{CO_2} values measured with electrodes maintained at 37°C to the patient's body temperature.

Howell et al. [11] and Rahn et al. [4] have shown that in vivo changes in P_{CO_2} and pH in ectotherms, which change body temperature with ambient temperature, are very similar to in vitro changes that take place in an anaerobic sample that is cooled [11, 33]. Evidence has been presented by Rahn et al. [4] that suggests that the correct intracellular pH during cooling is the pH of electrochemical neutrality of water (where pH = pOH), which is 6.80 at 37°C, with body fluids maintained at 0.6–0.8 pH units to the alkaline side of this. Since the pH of electrochemical neutrality of water rises as the temperature falls, the pH of body fluids should change by the same amount to maintain this difference. As mentioned earlier, under these conditions ionization of inter-mediate metabolic compounds remains maximal so that they cannot diffuse across cell membranes.

A wide range of cold-blooded vertebrates and invertebrates vary body pH in this way when acclimatized to different temperatures maintaining constant arterial CO_2 content [4]. It should be emphasized that, in poikilotherms as well as in homeotherms, it is the hydroxyl–hydrogen ion concentration ratio (OH^-/H^+) rather than the blood pH that is defended in normal acid–base regulation, so that a constant protein net charge of the intracellular compart-ment is preserved. Moreover, when these defense mechanisms are overcome by cold as hypothermia progresses in homeotherms, who do indeed protect blood pH levels at normothermia by renal and ventilatory adjustments, the blood buffer systems are released to defend the hydroxyl–hydrogen ion con-centration ratio and intracellular neutrality. In other words, the cell, whose acid–base status is that of neutrality for a given temperature, is bathed by extracellular fluid with a relative alkalinity. The extracellular environment acts as a sink to carry away the acid metabolites of the tissue, at the same time maintaining constant alkalinity relative to intracellular neutrality.

The difference between the pH of the extracellular environment and the pH of intracellular neutrality (pN) at all biological temperatures appears to be constant in a given species. Designated as K, the constant varies between 0.6 and 0.8 pH units. Thus, the pH of extracellular fluid is pN ± K. This relationship is achieved by the specific permeability and transport characteristics of the cell membrane. The buffering capacity of the extracellular fluid system involving the unique properties of the protein buffer, imidazole of histidine, and the precise regulation of the bicarbonate buffer ratio by proper ventilation and renal control help to maintain acid–base stability with changing temperature on both sides of the cell membrane. Actual in vivo observations of the behavior of human blood as it flows from heart to capillary and is cooled could be made by comparing pH of blood from skin capillary 25°C, heart 37°C, and exercising muscle 41°C. In this system, carbon dioxide content is fixed. Observed pH values of 7.60 in skin and 7.35 in muscle confirm that, in arterial blood of human beings, the OH^-/H^+ ratio has been held constant within this temperature range. It is important to note that the blood of humans, even when their core temperature is normothermic, has a spectrum of pH values. Its pH will depend upon where it is sampled if correction for temperature is to be made. Thus, 7.40 is not the only normal pH for human beings [34, 35], because, on a cold and windy day, an exercising person may exhibit local temperatures that may differ by a much as 20°C or more.

Homeotherms developed evolutionary mechanisms to defend both their temperature and their pH of 7.40 against any change. Through different physiologic mechanisms controlling the routing of blood to the periphery and initiating hypermetabolism, they fight to maintain homeothermy. If body temperature starts to fall, pH is protected by ventilatory regulation of CO_2 and renal regulations of HCO_3^- until exhaustion and death supervene. Because the buffer systems in the extracellular and intracellular compartment of humans and ectotherms are similar, it is advantageous to manage the patient as if he or she were a turtle. With thermoregulating mechanisms suppressed by anesthesia and both pulmonary- and renal acid–base-regulating mechanisms suppressed by both anesthesia and cold, during general hypothermia to a body temperature as low as 15°C, human beings appear to behave as poikilotherms. If ventilation is kept constant, the "internal milieu" of a patient will reveal the pH and P_{CO_2} curves shown in figure 4-4, where optimal conditions will be provided to preserve intracellular neutrality [4]. This requires that no CO_2 be added to the gas mixture. The rate and volume of each respiration should approximate those of normal alert breathing, which should create a moderate relative hyperventilation as metabolic CO_2 production is suppressed by cold. This should implement the desired fall in P_{CO_2} caused by increasing solubility

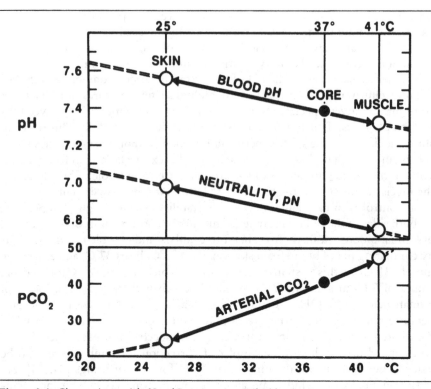

Figure 4-4. Changes in arterial pH and Pco_2 in man at 37°C blood arrives at the skin or exercising muscle at temperatures of 25°C and 41°C, respectively. Neutrality of water, pN, changes in parallel with changes in blood pH. Thus, the relative alkalinity of the blood, or the ratio between $(OH)^-$ and $(H)^+$ ions remains constant.

of CO_2 in association with the rise of pH induced by the changing ionization constant of water (Kw).

$$HOH \qquad H^+ + OH^-$$

$$\qquad Kw$$

The hydrogen ion concentration expressed in terms of pH and pOH has the following relationship relative to the neutral point of water:

$$pN = \frac{pH + pOH}{2} = \frac{1}{2} pKw$$

where pKw is the dissociation constant of water at a given temperature, pN is the pH of neutrality, and pOH is the approximate concentration of hydroxyl ions in a solution.

Constant ventilation during hypothermia was proposed by Severinghaus in 1959 [35]. Since then, however, concerns about cerebral blood flow and function have been expressed because of the decrease seen in cerebral blood flow associated with hypocarbia and normothermia [37]. However, this concern appears inappropriate in reference to Rahn's hypothesis applicable to hypothermia. Animal studies have shown that the reduction in blood flow with hypothermia is more nearly in 1:1 proportion to the reduction in whole body MR_{O_2} when minute ventilation is unchanged during cooling [38]. Moreover, it has been demonstrated that cerebral metabolism remains aerobic with equivalent decreases in P_{CO_2} versus temperature. Evidence suggests that the response of cerebral blood flow to P_{CO_2} is shifted appropriately with temperature. Cerebral ischemia is therefore unlikely when the uncorrected pH and P_{CO_2} values are normal. Another argument against using uncorrected values as a guide concerns changes in the oxyhemoglobin dissociation curve with temperature and pH. As the temperature decreases, the curve shifts to the left. The same shift occurs with an increase in the pH. It could be assumed that a combination of low body temperature and high pH might seem to be deleterious to tissue oxygen supply. However, evidence of problems with tissue oxygenation have not been proclaimed and it appears equally likely that offsetting changes in hemoglobin affinity compensate for the apparent shifts in the dissociation curve.

The effect of temperature on both the solubility of oxygen in plasma and the affinity of hemoglobin for oxygen makes temperature correction of measured oxygen tensions in the blood a complex matter. Complete saturation of hemoglobin with oxygen can be assumed regardless of temperature when P_{O_2} is 250 mmHg or greater [39].

Adding CO_2 to keep the corrected pH near 7.40 resulted in significant ventilatory effort in man under anesthesia [40]. With an understanding of the nature of the decrease in cerebral blood flow, it appears that constant minute ventilation (and hence constant uncorrected pH) is preferable. Further support for this is given by Becker et al. [41], who clearly showed in an experimental animal model that, where pH was increased during cooling, myocardial performance after ischemia was normal, as compared with a control group where pH was maintained at 7.40 in whom there was marked myocardial damage.

Keeping pH at 7.40 and Pa_{CO_2} at 38 mmHg at 22°C caused cerebral blood flow during surface cooling to fall 75% while raising pH to 7.75 and lowering Pa_{CO_2} to 10 mmHg allowed twice as much cerebral blood flow. By maintaining a pH of 7.40 not corrected for temperature during hypothermic cardiopulmonary bypass, Matthews et al. [42] have noticed higher perfusion pressures in the patient, together with urine excretion, even at 20°C, and no cerebral complications attributable to the change in technique. They proclaim that acid–base status remains stable, metabolic acidosis gradually diminishes, and additional sodium bicarbonate is no longer required at the end of bypass. According to these authors, cardiac dysrhythmias are less common, serum potassium remains stable, and myocardial contractility at the end of bypass in uncomplicated cases is such that inotropic support is unnecessary.

Work done in the early 1950s on hpothermia without cardiopulmonary by-pass led Virtue [43] to state that "a low carbon dioxide content and a high pH of the blood are desirable but further documentation of this factor is necessary." This statement was based on the information that spontaneous ventricular fibrillation was less of a problem when the pH was kept high. As Rahn et al. [4] have proposed, this situation maintains constant ionic charges on active protein molecules, thus possibly optimizing enzyme function. Studies done by Swain et al. [44] demonstrate that allowing the pH to rise with hypothermia and remain alkalotic relative to pH 7.40 improves the electrical stability of the heart during hypothermia, as evidenced by the VF threshold at 25°C. Since the ectothermic scheme increases the electrical stability of the heart, it could decrease the incidence of VF during hypothermia and decrease the temperature at which VF occurs during hypothermic cardiopulmonary bypass.

BEHAVIOR OF HUMAN BLOOD IN VITRO

When blood temperature is changed in a closed system, such as a syringe, in which only heat can exchange with the external environment, plasma pH and P_{CO_2} undergo marked changes. In contrast, the distribution between cells and plasma of Cl^- and HCO_3^- and red cell volume remain constant. During cooling, although the H^+ concentration decreases, the relative alkalinity (i.e., the difference between blood pH and pH of neutral water at the same tempera-ture) is preserved. CO_2 tension decreases, not only because of increases in its solubility and changes in pK of the bicarbonate buffer system, but also because of the increase in pH [15]. The temperature relationships of pH and log P_{CO_2} are fairly nonlinear, but can be accurately accounted for by a single-phase binary buffer system, composed of CO_2–bicarbonate and protein imidazole of histidine [3, 7]. At all temperatures, the net charge of the imidazole buffer, like the OH^-/H^+ ratio, remains constant.

ACID–BASE EQUILIBRA DURING HYPOTHERMIA IN MAN

In most in vivo situations, blood is not a closed but an open system because it is continuously exchanging gases, water, solutes, and heat with alveolar gas, renal fluids, or other surrounding tissues. Accordingly, it is difficult to define a normal acid–base state when blood pH and P_{CO_2} are affected simultaneously by temperature and by metabolic and/or respiratory variations.

In such an open system, pH and P_{CO_2} values depend on alveolar ventilation relative to CO_2 production. As stated, Rahn's hypothesis is that, at any body temperature and its associated metabolic rate, ventilation is normally adjusted to preserve a constant relative alkalinity and constant net charge of the imida-zole buffer [4]. During hypothermia, this requires that arterial P_{CO_2} decrease [11, 25]. Both protein buffer concentration (i.e., hemoglobin concentration) and hematocrit remain constant during hypothermia. Moreover, because buffers were not administered, it can be concluded from the normal values of pH at 37°C (7.40 ± 0.04) that nonrespiratory acidosis is absent during hypothermia.

Acid–base equilibrium during hypothermia, shown in the values of mixed venous blood, also proves that the behavior of human blood is the same in vivo as in vitro. Because CO_2 content remained constant, a pH value that ensured a constant OH^-/H^+ ratio is maintained during the cooling phase.

ADEQUACY OF OXYGENATION DURING HYPOTHERMIA

Cellular metabolic needs for oxygen, which are particularly temperature and pH dependent, are satisfied when O_2 availability exceeds O_2 utilization. Regardless of temperature, the availability of O_2 is determined by cardiac output (or blood perfusion pressure during extracorporeal bypass), regional blood flow, arterial Po_2 and O_2 content, and oxyhemoglobin dissociation. During hypothermia, there are several factors that can act in concert to decrease tissue Po_2. Thus, even though O_2 consumption is lower during hypothermia than during normothermia, cellular hypoxia may theoretically result from one or more of the following: (a) The leftward shift in the oxyhemoglobin dissociation curve. At 27°C, P_{50} is approximately 16.5 mmHg for neutral conditions (pH 7.55 and Pco_2 24 mmHg) [45]; accordingly, tissue Po_2 must decrease at any given So_2. (b) The decreased rate of oxyhemoglobin chemical equilibrium [46]. During hypothermia, therefore, at the prevailing regional Po_2, less O_2 may be released during the brief time that red blood cells spend in tissue capillaries. (c) The decreased rate of molecular diffusion. Thus, for a given concentration difference and pathway length, diffusion is slower in cool than in warm tissues.

Despite these minor considerations, however, evidence suggests that the low $\dot{V}o_2$ values during hypothermia [47, 48] are adequate to satisfy the patients O_2 requirements: (a) Arteriovenous O_2 difference is decreased during hypothermia; this means that total perfusion remains high relative to overall $\dot{V}o_2$. (b) Mixed venous Po_2, which can be viewed as the lowest mean effective Po_2 in the transport of O_2 from the bloodstream to average tissue, increases during hypothermia and returns (decreases) to normal values with rewarming. (c) Splanchnic Po_2, which has been shown to reflect the relationships between splanchnic perfusion and local $\dot{V}o_2$ [49], was greater than mixed venous Po_2. (d) Finally, the absence of metabolic acidosis excludes the presence of sufficient anaerobic metabolism to cause retention of organic acids in the blood.

Change in Po_2 in a closed system

The Po_2 of whole blood is a function of oxygen solubility and hemoglobin affinity for oxygen [50]. As the solubility of oxygen increases (with decreasing temperature), the Po_2 declines. The change of Po_2 with respect to temperature depends on the degree that hemoglobin is saturated with oxygen. The affinity of hemoglobin for oxygen at 0°C is 22-fold more than at 37°C, but the solubility of oxygen (in water) is only doubled. Therefore, as blood is cooled, the Po_2 decreases, owing to increased solubility. Hemoglobin more avidly binds oxygen, causing the Po_2 to decrease further. This shift of dissolved oxygen to bound oxygen is small compared with the amount of oxygen previously bound; therefore, the degree of saturation does not change significantly.

Myocardial damage caused by keeping pH 7.40 during systemic deep hypothermia

Becker et al. [41] carried out a study on puppy hearts that was designed to test the hypothesis that application of the ectothermal strategy for pH and Pco_2 adjustment during deep levels of immersion and perfusion hypothermia (17°C) would allow (a) better myocardial performance and organ perfusion during cooling and (b) better cardiac recovery after a standard 60-min interval of circulatory arrest with "ideal" cardioplegic protection. They had previously shown that the bypassed heart functions better at 28°C if pH is adjusted to ectothermic levels [51]. It was found that constraining pH to 7.40 during surface hypothermia reproduced the profound depression in cardiac output, cerebral and coronary blood flow, lactic acidosis, and ultimate ventricular fibrillation reported by others [52]. Repeated defibrillations were necessary for cardiac resuscitation during rewarming and reperfusion, and postischemic recovery of left ventricular performance was incomplete. In contrast, applying the strategy for pH management used by cold–blooded animals (ectotherms) allowed better maintenance of cardiac output and organ perfusion during cooling and prevented lactic acidosis and ventricular fibrillation. Regular cardiac rhythm resumed spontaneously during rewarming and myocardial performance recovered completely.

Blood pH 7.40 at 37°C, therefore, is alkaline to the 6.80 neutral point of water at that temperature. It is recognized from physical chemistry that the neutral point of water is temperature dependent and rises as temperature falls because of changes in its ionization constant [53]. Water pH must rise from 6.80 to 7.40 to maintain neutrality if water temperature is lowered from 37°C to 3°C. Similarly, blood pH should increase with hypothermia according to the concept of Peters and Van Slyke [12], who in 1932 stated "that for the maintenance of the organism in a state compatible with life, the reaction of the inner fluids must be slightly to the alkaline side of the neutral point and that much deviation from this physiologic reaction is disastrous."

In 1948, Rosenthal [14] reported similar physical chemical behavior of in vitro mammalian blood samples held in gas-tight syringes where a Δ pH/°C = 0.015 occurs when measurements in an enclosed electrode system are made at various temperatures. This correction factor is used in clinical blood gas laboratories where blood samples taken from hypothermic patients are warmed to 37°C for analysis and results are reported as measured (meter) and corrected values. For example, a blood sample from a patient at 17°C, measured at 37°C, will have a pH meter value of 7.10, but will be reported as a corrected value of 7.40.

In 1970, Howell and associates [11] reported a widespread in vivo phylogenetic adherence to the principle of relative alkalinity by measuring arterial pH in cold-blooded animals at different body temperatures. In these animals, carbon dioxide is reduced to keep pH alkaline to the neutral point of water. The only exception to this rule seems to be hibernating mammals, in which pH regularly stays at 7.40 over a wide temperature range [53] [54] while the animals hypoventilate with hypothermia. The importance of the ectothermic approach to pH and P_{CO_2} management was recognized by Swan [55] in 1974. One year later Rahn et al. [4] focused clinical attention on Howell's observation in ectotherms by pointing out that an entire spectrum of vertebrates and invertebrates follow a thermal pattern whereby pH rises as temperature falls to maintain relative alkalinity. They showed that this change was due to the dominant effect of protein buffers, principally the imidazole of histidine. The pH was raised by reducing carbon dioxide and it was shown that the best myocardial performance at 28°C occurred at pH 7.72, where left ventricular blood flow, oxygen, and lactate metabolism were greatest. This pH correction is at the higher limits of the pH range reported in ectotherms and served as a basis for the correction factor.

CURRENT PRACTICE

Most blood gas laboratories measure pH at 37°C, and clinical pH management during hypothermia follows one of three regimens. *First,* if pH 7.40 is considered ideal and the correction factor is either not applied or not reported, gas mixtures are adjusted by the anesthesiologist or perfusionist to keep this value. It should be recognized that the true pH (temperature corrected) is higher and in the proper direction from a phylogenetic point of view. *Second,* if there is awareness of the correction factor and a similar adherence to keeping pH 7.40, P_{CO_2} will be altered to achieve this level during hypothermia. For example, a 27°C, pH 7.55 blood sample analyzed at 37°C would be reported as pH 7.40 uncorrected at 37°C and pH 7.55 corrected. Under these circumstances, carbon dioxide would be added to achieve a corrected reading of 7.40 at 27°C. This would be an acidotic pH for an ectotherm and a departure from the ideal suggested by Peters and Van Slyke [12]. However, this is the pattern practiced by hibernating animals and perhaps the most commonly used pH management in clinical practice. *Third,* pH may be varied to produce relative alkalosis either by adjusting P_{CO_2} [56, 57] or by adding fixed base (i.e., $NaHCO_3$ or trimethamine) [58]. The concept of inducing respiratory alkalosis during hypothermia was introduced by Mohri and associates [56] several years ago and used by McDonnell and associates [51] since 1975 to achieve an even greater degree of relative alkalosis. Carbon dioxide regulation to produce the desired pH during hypothermia carries the advantages of (a) following phylogenetic strategy, (b) ensuring rapid entry into the cell and immediate buffering, and, (c) easier regulation during rewarming to avoid persistent metabolic alkalosis when pH 7.40 is desirable [58].

Studies done by Becker et al. [41] during surface cooling showed that systolic blood pressure and cardiac indices were maintained better when pH was manipulated to produce a level at the upper (alkalotic) range of ectotherms under similar temperatures. In contrast, keeping pH 7.40 (corrected for temperature) resulted in a substantial fall in circulatory indices and metabolic evidence of inadequate cardiac output; systemic lactic acidosis developed in the same way as reported in clinical and experimental studies [52, 59–61]. In comparison, systemic lactate metabolism remained normal when pH was adjusted to produce more relative alkalinity. The principle cause for better cardiac performance during surface cooling in pH-adjusted dogs was a more ideal biochemical environment for continued aerobic metabolism; left ventricular oxygen uptake per beat increased progressively and no myocardial lactate production or ventricular fibrillation occurred. Conversely, a less ideal biochemical environment was evident during surface cooling in non-pH-adjusted dogs; subendocardial blood flow was less well maintained, myocardial lactate production occurred at 22°C, and ventricular fibrillation developed in all dogs at or before 22°C was reached. The findings by Becker et al. [41] were consistent with those of Rittenhouse and colleagues [57], who avoided ventricular fibrillation by producing moderate respiratory alkalosis during surface cooling to as low as 19°C. They imposed more pronounced respiratory alkalosis and observed less fall in cardiac indices at low temperatures. Other causes for better cardiac performance include the inotropic effect of respiratory alkalosis [62] which might have been added to the inotropic effect of hypothermia itself [63, 64]. This explanation is supported by the increased myocardial oxygen consumption per beat in pH-adjusted dogs. On the basis of the concept of relative alkalosis, pH 7.40 would be considered acidotic during hypothermia. The importance of avoiding intracellular acidosis during hypothermia is emphasized by studies by Poole-Wilson and Langer [65], showing profound negative inotropic effect of respiratory acidosis at 24°C.

CEREBRAL PERFUSION

In the past, there has been some reluctance to produce alkalosis by hyperventilation owing to the concern of cerebral hypoperfusion during hypocapnia at 37°C [66].

However, data obtained by Becker et al. [41] show that total and regional brain blood flow (cerebrum, brain stem, cerebellum) was maintained better (25% below control values) in pH-adjusted dogs despite lowering of P_{CO_2} to 10 mmHg at 22°C. Conversely, the marked cerebral hypoperfusion (75% below control values) produced by keeping pH 7.40 (corrected for temperature) was similar to that reported by others when higher P_{CO_2} levels were maintained [67–69]. It has been proposed that maintenance of higher systemic blood pressure and cardiac index allowed more adequate cerebral perfusion and that cerebral vasoregulation may have functioned better in the alkaline pH environment. The potential benefits of lowering P_{CO_2} and keeping pH higher during hypothermia are supported by the studies reported by Norwood et al. [70], showing that such pH manipulations significantly ameliorate the no reflow lesions seen after anoxic cold brain perfusion. The profound cerebral hypoperfusion at pH 7.40 during surface cooling calls attention to the role of cerebral ischemia before circulatory arrest in causing postoperative neurologic problems.

Systemic vascular resistance was 90% higher ($p < 0.05$) in the pH 7.40 studies than in those where more alkaline pH was maintained when hypothermic perfusion began at 80 mmHg to lower body temperature to 17°C. Assuming that the lowered resistance was shared by all organs, then pH adjustment with perfusion hypothermia may allow more rapid and homogeneous organ cooling and avoid the need for surface cooling where blood pressure and cardiac output decreases despite pH adjustment. Appropriate pH will not only stabilize the Gibbs–Donnan ratio and red blood cell volume, but will also prevent relative intracellular acidosis that can result in cellular swelling [4]. Reports of increasing hematocrit during hypothermia [71] without pH adjustment may be explained on this basis, and such swelling may limit the effectiveness of hemodilution and contribute to the impaired organ perfusion occurring with deeper levels of surface hypothermia. The completeness of recovery in all hearts subjected to pH adjustment suggests that myocardial cardioplegic protection was excellent. Conversely, failure of complete recovery in pH 7.40 experimental animals indicates that failure to provide pH adjustment was responsible for the damage. Systemic lactic acidosis developed in all dogs during circulatory arrest, so that pH was low during the initial phase of rewarming despite a reversal of the pattern of pH regulation. Systemic vascular resistance was 30% ($p < 0.05$) lower when cardiopulmonary bypass was restarted in the pH 7.40 group, presumably because more acid metabolites accumulated in these dogs; base excess recovered more slowly in them. Acid–base balance was restored when postischemic ventricular performance was tested 30 min later. Normally, regular sinus rhythm resumed spontaneously in dogs protected by multidose blood cardioplegia, and this occurred in five of six dogs in the pH-adjusted group. Conversely, each pH 7.40 dog had ventricular fibrillation during reperfusion, and repeated defibrillations were necessary before regular rhythm was established (averaging 14 min). The persistence of ventricular fibrillation during the early phases of rewarming may have contributed to the myocardial depression seen 30 min later.

Left ventricular performance returned to preischemic level in all dogs in which pH adjustment was imposed. Conversely, 50% depression of postischemic performance occurred in hearts receiving the same cardioplegic protection where pH was kept 7.40.

The slope for ideal pH for human hearts during hypothermia is unknown, but it has been shown that high-level mammalian hearts function better in the more alkalotic range when they are introduced into the realm of hypothermia.

Currently, pH values are reported as corrected readings only, rather than as meter readings at 37°C as they were several years ago. Consequently, a corrected pH of 7.40 during deep hypothermia would reflect a very profound relative acidosis. Studies by Halasz et al. [72] show that cold preservation of rabbit and canine kidneys at pHs in the alkaline range of 7.40 results in better recovery of function and less lysozymal enzyme release.

It can be concluded from the study done by Becker and associates in 1981 [41] that pH 7.40 may be neither normal nor ideal during hypothermia. Constraining pH to 7.40 during hypothermia causes a degree of myocardial damage and limitation of myocardial protection that are avoidable by pH adjustment to a position of relative alkalinity, as it occurs in ectotherms during cooling and rewarming. These findings may have major implications in the routine management of hypothermia during all cardiac operations.

In our institution, "uncorrected" values of pH and Pco_2 are used. If the measurements at 30°C in the electrode are in the normal range (i.e., pH = 7.40 ± 0.04 and Pco_2 = 40 ± 4.0 mmHg), we are satisfied that the patient's acid–base status is acceptable, and any adjustments are based on "uncorrected" values irrespective of the patient's actual temperature. Blayo et al. [73] recently confirmed this approach in patients undergoing cardiac surgery with hypothermia.

With thermoregulating mechanisms suppressed by anesthesia during hypothermia, human beings appear to behave as poikilotherms. The present study was designed to examine this statement.

Methods

A total of 34 patients (23 men and 11 women) 41–85 years old (mean, 64) who underwent open-heart surgery with hypothermia were studied. Anesthesia was induced with fentanyl (10–20 μg/kg) or sufentanil (2.0–5.0 μg/kg). Pancuronium bromide (0.1–0.15 mg/kg) was used to achieve muscle relaxation. Anesthesia was maintained with supplemental doses of fentanyl (50–100 μg), sufentanil (25 μg), or with a combination of a narcotic and a volatile agent such as halothane or isoflurane (0.5%–1.0%). Extracorporeal blood perfusion (ECBP) was performed with a roller pump and a membrane oxygenator. Initially, a cardiac index equal to 2.5 L/min/m² was maintained. During hypothermia, this was decreased to 1.8–2.2 L/min/m². The oxygenator gas mixture was adjusted as needed to keep arterial and venous blood gases within the normal range as measured at 37°C (not corrected for temperature). Buffers were not administered during bypass. By controlling the temperature of the perfusate, core temperature was reduced to 25°–30°C. The myocardium was protected by intermittent perfusion of a cold blood cardioplegic solution containing 60 meq kCl so that myocardial temperature during clamping was less than 20°C. Rewarming was started once the aorta was unclamped. Blood gases were determined before bypass, during hypothermia, and after bypass using an ABL-1 (radio-meter) blood gas machine.

Statistical analysis

HCO_3^-, pH, P_{CO_2}, and mixed venous O_2 data for each period examined are shown in the table 4-1. All results are expressed as the mean value and standard error of the mean. A paired t-test, with p values obtained from the Student-Fisher table was employed to determine the difference between the results at different periods. Pre- and postbypass P_{CO_2} values were not significantly different ($p < 0.05$), and pH and HCO_3^- values remained constant at all temperatures.

Results

Initially, slight hypocapnia with moderate reduction in HCO_3^- content was observed due to excessive ventilation at the beginning of surgery with a pH value of 7.42 ± 0.6. Normal pH values (7.45 ± 0.8) were obtained during ECBP with hypothermia (table 4-1). During the rewarming process, the pH values were 7.40 ± 0.7. Constant pH values measured at 37°C prove that a constant OH^-/H^+ ratio was present at all temperatures. Prebypass Pa_{CO_2} was 35.2 ± 7.8 mmHg, which remained at a steady level of 36.0 ± 5.0 mmHg during the hypothermic bypass period and was equal to 35.0 ± 8.0 mmHg during the rewarming process. The prebypass value of HCO_3^- was 22.3 ± 4.4 meq/L, which went up to a value of 24.4 ± 2.9 meq/L during the period of hypothermic bypass and returned to a value of 22.6 ± 2.3 meq/L for the rewarming period (figure 4-5). Because the bicarbonate concentration and total CO_2 content (T_{CO_2}) remained unchanged during hypothermia, acidosis due to nonvolatile acid production can be excluded. Furthermore, a significant buffer concentration difference could not be found either before, during, or after ECBP. In none of the patients studied was the mixed $P\bar{V}_{O_2}$ less than 45 mmHg, suggesting adequate tissue perfusion during hypothermia.

Discussion

Actual in vivo observations of the behavior of human blood as it flows from heart to capillary and is cooled can be made by comparing pH of blood from skin capillary 25°C, heart 37°C, and exercising muscle 41°C. Observed pH values of 7.60 in skin and 7.35 in muscle would confirm that, in arterial blood

Table 4-1. Data for each period examined

	Prebypass 35°–37°C	Hypothermia 25°–30°C	Postbypass 35°–37°C
pH	7.42 ± 0.06	7.45 ± 0.08	7.40 ± 0.07
Pa_{CO_2}	35.2 ± 7.8	36.0 ± 5.0	35.0 ± 8.0
$P\bar{V}_{O_2}$	52.3 ± 5.6	58.0 ± 10.0	51.8 ± 7.0
HCO_3^-	22.3 ± 4.4	24.4 ± 2.9	22.6 ± 2.3

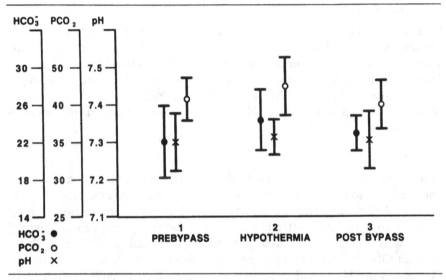

Figure 4-5. Graphic representation of the mean values of (HCO_3^-), P_{CO_2}, and pH during the prebypass and postbypass periods and during hypothermia. The *vertical lines* represent 1 standard deviation. All measurements were made at 37°C.

of human beings, the OH^-/H^+ ratio has been held constant within this temperature range. This allows us to conclude that human blood, even when core temperature is normothermic, has a spectrum of pH values. If ventilation is kept constant, the "internal milieu" of a patient will reveal specific pH and P_{CO_2} curves, where optimal conditions will be provided to preserve intracellular neutrality. This requires that no CO_2 be added to the gas mixture. Constant ventilation during hypothermia was proposed in 1959. Animal studies have shown that the reduction in cerebral blood flow with hypothermia is in 1:1 proportion to the reduction in whole body MR_{O_2} when minute ventilation is unchanged during cooling. Keeping pH at 7.40 and Pa_{CO_2} at 38 mmHg at 22°C caused cerebral blood flow during surface cooling to fall 75% while raising pH to 7.75 and lowering Pa_{CO_2} to 10 mmHg allowed twice as much cerebral blood flow. Literature data also indicate that, when pH was increased during cooling, myocardial performance after ischemia was normal, as compared with a control group where, when pH was maintained at 7.40 (corrected for temperature), there was marked myocardial damage. Our data demonstrate that, by maintaining a pH of 7.40 (not corrected for temperature) during hypothermia, the acid–base status remains stable, cardiac dysrhythmias are less common, and myocardial contractility at the end of bypass in uncomplicated cases is such that inotropic support becomes less necessary. It has been proposed that cerebral vasoregulation may function better in the alkaline pH environment. The potential benefits of lowering P_{CO_2} and keeping pH higher during hypothermia are supported by many authors showing that such pH manipulations significantly ameliorate the *no reflow lesions* seen after anoxic cold brain perfusion.

REFERENCES

1. Davis BD: On the importance of being ionized. Arch Biochem Biophys 78:497, 1958.
2. Burton RF: The role of buffers in body fluids: mathematical analysis. Respir Physiol 18: 34–42, 1973.
3. Reeves RB: Temperature induced changes in blood acid–base status: pH and P_{CO_2} in a binary buffer. J Appl Physiol 40:752–761, 1976.
4. Rahn H, Reeves RB, Howell BJ: Hydrogen ion regulation, temperature, and evolution. Am Rev Respir Dis 112:165–172, 1975.
5. Reeves RB, Wilson TL: Intracellular pH in bullfrog striated and cardiac muscle as a function of body temperature. Fed Proc 28:782, 1969.
6. Malan A, Reeves RB: Intracellular pH in turtles (*Pseudemys scripta*) tissues as a function of body temperature. Physiologist 16:385, 1973.
7. Reeves RB: An imidazole alphastat hypothesis for vertebrate acid–base regulation: tissue carbon dioxide content and body temperature in bullfrogs. Respir Physiol 14:219–236, 1972.
8. Reeves RB: Temperature induced changes in whole blood pH and P_{CO_2} at constant carbon dioxide content. Fed Proc 32:349, 1973.
9. Reeves RB, Malan A: Model studies in intracellular acid–base temperature responses in ectotherms. Respir Physiol 28:49–63, 1976.
10. Rahn H: Body temperature and acid–base regulation. Pneumonologic 151:87–97, 1974.
11. Howell BJ, Baumgardner FW, Bondi K, et al.: Acid–base balance in cold blood vertebrates as a function of body temperature. Am J Physiol 218:600–606, 1970.
12. Peters JP, Van Slyke DD: Quantitative clinical chemistry. Williams and Wilkins, Baltimore, 1932, pp 245 and 868.
13. Robin ED: Relationship between temperature and plasma pH and carbon dioxide tension in the turtle. Nature 195:249–250 1962.
14. Rosenthal TB: The effects of temperature on the pH of the blood and plasma in vitro. J Biol Chem 173:25–30, 1948.
15. Rahn H: P_{CO_2}, pH and body temperature. In: Nahas GG, Schaefer KE (eds) Carbon dioxide and metabolic regulation. Springer-Verlag, Berlin, 1974, pp 151–162.
16. Reeves RB: Temperature-induced changes in blood–base status: Donnan r_{Cl} red cell volume. J Appl Physiol 40:762–767, 1976.
17. Rahn H: Gas transport from the external environment to the cell. In: de Revch Avs, Porter R (eds) Development of the lung. Ciba Foundation symposium. J and A Churchill, London, 1966, pp 3–23.
18. Jackson DC: The effect of temperature on ventilation in the turtle, *Pseudemys scripta elegans*. Respir Physiol 12:131–140, 1971.
19. Jackson DC, Palmer SE, Meadow WL: The effects of temperature and carbon dioxide breathing on ventilation and acid–base status of turtles. Respir Physiol 20:131–146, 1974.
20. Davies DG, Kopetzky MT: Effect of body temperature on the ventilatory response to hypercapnia in the awake alligator. Fed Proc 35:840, 1976.
21. Jackson DC, Silverblatt H: Respiration and acid–base status of turtles following experimental dives. Am J Physiol 226:903–909, 1974.
22. Alberry WJ, Lloyd BB: Variation of chemical potential with temperature. In: de Reuch AVS, Porter R (eds) Development of the lung. Little, Brown, and Company, Boston, 1967, pp 30–33.
23. Malan A, Wilson TL, Reeves RB: Intracellular pH in cold-blooded vertebrates as a function of body temperature. Respir Physiol 28:29–47, 1976.
24. Wood SC, Moberly WR: The influence of temperature on the respiratory properties of iguana blood. Respir Physiol 10:20–29, 1970.
25. Rahn H, Baumgardner FW: Temperature and acid–base regulation in fish. Respir Physiol 14: 171–182, 1972.
26. Nunn JF: Applied respiratory physiology, 2nd edn. Butterworths, London, 1977, p 347.

27. Kelman GR, Nunn JF: Nomograms for correction of blood Po_2, Pco_2, pH, and base excess for time and temperature. J Appl Physiol 21:1490, 1966.
28. Siggard-Andersen O: Titrable acid or base of body fluids. Ann NY Acad Sci 133:41–58, 1966.
29. Severinghaus JW, Stuppel M, Bradley AF: Accuracy of blood pH and Pco_2 determinations. J Appl Physiol 9:189–196, 1956.
30. Severinghaus JW, Stuppel M, Bradley AF: Variations of serum carbonic acid pK' and pH with temperature. J Appl Physiol 9:297–300, 1956.
31. Nunn JF, Bergman NA, Bunatyan A, Coleman AJ: Temperature coefficients for Pco_2 and Po_2 of blood in vitro. J Appl Physiol 20:23–26, 1965.
32. Gershwin R, Smith NT, Suwa K: An equation system and programs for obtaining base excess using a programmable calculator. Anesthesiology 40:89–92, 1974.
33. Rahn H: Acid–base regulation and temperature in the evolution of verebrates. Proc Int Union Physiol Sci 8:91–92, 1971.
34. Swan H: The hydroxyl–hydrogen ion concentration ratio during hypothermia. Surg Gynecol Obstet 155:897–912, 1982.
35. Ream AK, Reitz BA, Silverberg G: Temperature correction of Pco_2 and pH in estimating acid–base status: an example of the emperor's new clothes? Anesthesiology 56:41–44, 1982.
36. Severinghaus JW: Respiration and hypothermia. Ann NY Acad Sci 80:384–394, 1959.
37. Hagerdal M, Harp JR, Siesjo BK: Influence of changes in arterial Pco_2 on cerebral blood flow and cerebral energy state during hypothermia in the rat. Acta Anaesth Scand [Suppl] 57: 25–33, 1975.
38. Ohmura AA, Wong KC, Westenskow DR: Effects of hypocarbia and normocarbia on cardiovascular dynamics and regional circulation in the hypothermic dog. Anesthesiology 50:293–298, 1979.
39. Hedley-Whyte J: O_2 solubility in blood and temperature correction factors for Po_2. J Appl Physiol 19:901–906, 1964.
40. Carson SAA, Morris LE: Controlled acid–base status with cardiopulmonary bypass and hypothermia. Anesthesiology 23:618–626, 1962.
41. Becker H, Vinton-Johnsen J, Buckberg GD, et al.: Myocardial damage caused by keeping pH 7.40 during systemic deep hypothermia. J Thorac Cardiovasc Surg 82:810–820, 1981.
42. Matthews AJ, Stead AL, Abbott TR: Acid–base control during hypothermia. Anaesthesia 39:649–654, 1984.
43. Virtue RW: Hypothermia anesthesia. Charles C Thomas, Springfield IL, 1955, p 54.
44. Swain JA, White RN, Peters RM: The effect of pH on the hypothermic ventricular fibrillation threshold. J Thorac Cardiovasc Surg 87:445–451, 1984.
45. Castaing M, Pocidaly JJ: Temperature and acid–base status of human blood at constant and variable total CO_2 content. Respir Physiol 38:243–256, 1979.
46. Roughton FJW: Transport of oxygen and carbon dioxide. In: Fern WO, Rahn H (eds) Handbook of physiology, sect 3, Respiration, vol 1. American Physiological Society, Washington DC, 1964, pp 767–825.
47. Abott TR: Oxygen uptake following deep hypothermia. Anesthesia 32:524–532, 1977.
48. Lunding M, Rygg IH: Evaluation of the sufficiency of tissue oxygenation during cardiopulmonary bypass and hypothermia. Scand J Thorac Cardiovasc Surg 2:169–178, 1968.
49. Pocidalo JJ, Vallois JM, Martinelli J, et al.: Po_2 et Pco_2 d'un liquide artificiel tonométrédans la cavite peritoneale: correlations avec le sang veineux portal. J Physiol (Paris) 67:214A, 1973.
50. Ashwood ER, Kost G, Kenny M: Temperature correction of blood-gas and pH measurements. Clin Chem 29:1877–1885, 1983.
51. McConnell DH, White F, Nelson R, et al.: Importance of alkalosis in maintenance of ideal blood pH during hypothermia. Surg Forum 26:263–265, 1975.
52. Shida H, Morimoto M, Inokawa K, et al.: Simple deep hypothermia for open-heart surgery. J Cardiovasc Surg 20:135, 1979.
53. Austin JH, Cullen GE: Hydrogen ion concentration of the blood in health and disease. Medicine 4:275, 1925.
54. Goodrich CA: Acid–base balance in euthermic and hibernating marmots. Am J Physiol 224: 1185–1189, 1973.
55. Swan H: Thermoregulation and bioenergetics: patterns for vertebrate survival. Elsevier, New York, 1974, pp 180–187.
56. Mohri H, Dillare DH, Crawford WE, et al.: Method of surface-induced deep hypothermia

for open-heart surgery in infants. J Thorac Cardiovasc Surg 58:262–271, 1969.

57. Rittenhouse EA, Ito CS, Mohri H, et al.: Circulatory dynamics during surface-induced deep hypothermia and after cardiac arrest for one hour. J Thorac Cardiovasc Surg 61:359, 1971.
58. Ellis RJ, Hoover E, Gay WA, et al.: Metabolic alterations with profound hypothermia. Arch Surg 109:659, 1974.
59. Johnston AE, Radde IC, Steward DJ, et al.: Acid–base and electrolyte changes in infants undergoing profound hypothermia for surgical correction of congenital heart defects. Can Anaesth Soc J 21:23, 1974.
60. Steward DJ, Sloan IA, Johnston AE: Anaesthetic management of infants undergoing profound hypothermia for surgical correction of congenital heart defects. Can Anaesth Soc J 21:15, 1974.
61. Bigelow WG, Callaghan JC, Hopps JA: General hypothermia for experimental intra-cardiac surgery: the use of electrophrenic respirations, an artifical pacemaker for cardiac stand-still and radio-frequency rewarming in general hypothermia. Ann Surg 132:531–539, 1950.
62. Streisand RL, Gourin A, Stuckey JH: Respiratory and metabolic alkalosis and myocardial contractility. J Thorac Cardiovasc Surg 620:431–438, 1971.
63. Buckberg GD, Brazier JR, Nelson RL, et al.: Studies of the effects of hypothermia on regional myocardial blood flow and metabolism during cardiopulmonary bypass. J Thorac Cardiovasc Surg 73:87, 1977.
64. Monroe RG, Strange RH, LaFarge CG, et al.: Ventricular performance pressure–volume relationship, and O_2 consumption during hypothermia. Am J Physiol 206:67, 1964.
65. Pole-Wilson PA, Langr GA: Effect of pH on ionic exchange and function in rat and rabbit myocardium. Am J Physiol 229:570, 1975.
66. Reivich M: Arterial P_{CO_2} and cerebral hemodynamics. Am J Physiol 206:25, 1964.
67. Kawashima U, Okada K, Kosugi I, et al.: Changes in distribution of cardiac output by surface-induced deep hypothermia in dogs. J Appl Physiol 40:876, 1976.
68. Su JY, Amory DW, Sands MP, et al.: Effects of ether anesthesia and surface induced hypothermia on regional blood flow. Am Heart J 97:53, 1979.
69. Rudy LW, Boucher JK, Edmunds LH: The effect of deep hypothermia and circulatory arrest on the distribution of system blood flow in rhesus monkeys. J Thorac Cardiovas Surg 64:706, 1972.
70. Norwood WJ, Norwood DR, Costaneda AR: Cerebral anoxia: effect of deep hypothermia and pH. Surgery 86:203, 1979.
71. Anzai T, Turner MD, Gibson WH, et al.: Blood flow distribution in dogs during hypothermia and posthypothermia. Am J Physiol 234:706, 1978.
72. Halasz NA, Collins GM, White FN: The right pH for preservation? In: Pegg D (ed) Organ preservation, vol 3. Churchill Livingstone, London, 1979, p 259.
73. Blayo MC, Lecompt Y, Pocidalo JJ: Control of acid–base status during hypothermia in man. Respir Physiol 42:287–298, 1980.

5. HIGH PUMP FLOWS AND PRESSURE ARE DESIRABLE DURING CARDIOPULMONARY BYPASS

KETAN SHEVDE
SARADA MYLAVARAPU

Cardiopulmonary bypass (CPB) is an essential part of the vast majority of cardiac surgical procedures. The main purpose of CPB is to provide adequate organ perfusion while maintaining a quiet, bloodless field during cardiac surgery after the application of an aortic cross clamp. This allows the surgeons to operate efficiently and expeditiously. Cardiac surgery is associated with a variety of postoperative complications such as myocardial ischemia, myocardial infarction [1, 2], ischemic brain injury [3], renal failure [4], pancreatic dysfunction [5], and ischemic bowel syndrome [6]. To what extent these undesirable effects are directly attributable to CPB is not always easy to determine. For example, when a patient develops neurologic dysfunction or renal failure after a prolonged and difficult operative procedure, it is unclear whether these complications are related to CPB, or low cardiac output syndrome, or the use of vasoactive pharmacologic agents. Prolonged low cardiac output states requiring the use of vasoconstrictor drugs presumably play a major role in the genesis of these undesirable complications. The maintenance of adequate perfusion pressure and flow rate during CPB is often dictated by experience accumulated from studies that are not necessarily performed on extracorporeal circulation. We will therefore refer to some studies not performed on CPB. Even when postoperative morbidity and mortality are directly related to CPB, it is more often due to air and/or particulate matter emboli than to low perfusion pressure or low flow. Frequently, neurologic complications are related to the type of surgical procedure. These complications are seen more frequently following valvular surgery than after aortocoronary bypass surgery [7], the implication being that air and particulate emboli are much more likely to result when the myocardial cavity is exposed to the atmosphere.

The advantages of low perfusion pressure and flow on CPB are generally considered to be minimal trauma to blood components, lower risk of tubing and connector failure, and decreased collateral flow to the left ventricle. However, there are several clinical entities where low pressure and low flow may prove to be detrimental to the patient. Specifically, these areas are:

1. Reduced oxygen-carrying capacity due to hemodilution and alkalosis
2. In patients with impending central nervous system dysfunction
3. Hypertension
4. In patients with coronary artery disease and generalized atherosclerosis.

In this chapter, the arbitrary levels of minimum blood pressure and flow rate are considered to be 50 mmHg and 1.5 L/min/m^2, respectively.

OXYGEN-CARRYING CAPACITY OF THE BLOOD DURING CPB

In order to have a better understanding of oxygen delivery during CPB, it is necessary to view the oxyhemoglobin dissociation curve, which has a well-documented sigmoid shape (figure 5-1). The curve corresponds to oxygen saturation at various levels of oxygen tension in the blood. The flat, top portion of the curve represents relatively high hemoglobin saturation, such that a decrease in arterial oxygen tension from 100 to 60 mmHg results in a modest 8% decline in hemoglobin saturation from 97% to 89%. Oxygen tension below 60 mmHg results in a steep decline in the hemoglobin saturation so that, at Po$_2$ of 40 mmHg, the hemoglobin saturation is only 75%. At normal pH, 50% hemoglobin saturation occurs at a Po$_2$ of ~27 mmHg. A convenient index of the affinity of hemoglobin for oxygen is P$_{50}$, described as the oxygen tension at which 50% of the hemoglobin is saturated. Using this index, one can refer to hemoglobin as in "holding on" to oxygen when P$_{50}$ declines, i.e., when the hemoglobin dissociation curve shifts to the left. Hemoglobin releases oxygen when P$_{50}$ increases, or when the curve shifts to the right. A number of factors can shift the curve to the right or to the left. For example, mild acidosis with a pH change from 7.4 to 7.2 can cause a 15% rightward shift of the curve and a mild alkalosis with pH change from 7.4 to 7.6 can cause an equivalent change in the opposite direction [8]. A decline in temperature causes a similar leftward shift to that of alkalosis. Both decrease in temperature and alkalosis are prevalent on CPB and are a major cause of decreased oxygen delivery to the tissues.

Another important factor to be considered is the use of stored blood during cardiac operative procedures. Stored blood has a decreased amount of 2, 3-diphosphoglycerate (2, 3-DPG), which shifts the hemoglobin dissociation

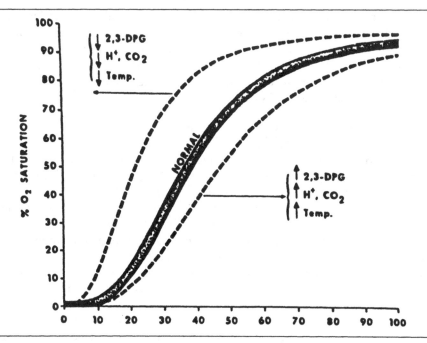

Figure 5-1. A schematic representation of the oxyhemoglobin dissociation curve showing the effect of 2, 3-diphosphoglycerate hydrogen iron (*2, 3-DPG*) concentration, CO_2 concentration, and *temperature* on the position of the curve.

curve to the left with resultant increase in affinity for oxygen [9]. Reduction in 2, 3-DPG occurs in both citrate phosphate dextrose (CPD) and citrate phosphate dextrose and adenine (CPDA) stored blood. Within days, the P_{50} and 2, 3-DPG values decreased from a normal of 26.5 mmHg and 4.8 µmol/ml to 18 mmHg and 1.2 µmol/ml, respectively, when stored in CPD solution [10]. Alkalosis and hypothermia cause a greater leftward shift of the curve than does decreased 2, 3-DPG. Both of these conditions are prevalent on CPB. Kawashima et al. have shown that there is a significant drop in oxygen consumption with a concomitant reduction in both arterial and venous O_2 content when the hematocrit decreases to less than 20% [11]. When the drop in hematocrit occurs over a number of days as in chronic anemia, there is a compensatory increase in 2, 3-DPG that shifts the oxyhemoglobin curve to the right to facilitate release of oxygen to the tissues.

This compensatory mechanism does not occur in patients undergoing CPB because hemodilution is almost instantaneous. In this situation, the oxygen-carrying capacity is drastically reduced and is exacerbated by alkalosis and decreased blood temperature, resulting in further diminution in oxygen delivery to the tissues. Litwak et al. have demonstrated that sudden hemodilution in the initial part of CPB can be well tolerated if high-flow total body perfusion is utilized [12]. It has been shown in animal experiments that the combination of decreased 2, 3-DPG, hypothermia, and alkalosis can result in a decrease in the myocardial performance, as evidenced by diminished stroke volume [13]. Moores showed that this decrease in myocardial performance was accompanied by a concomitant decrease in arterial-to-coronary sinus O_2 difference [14]. In order to compensate for these abberations in O_2 carrying capacity, high perfusion pressures and flow would seem beneficial.

CENTRAL NERVOUS SYSTEM DYSFUNCTION FOLLOWING CARDIOPULMONARY BYPASS

The diagnosis of brain dysfunction utilizing electroencephalogram (EEG) is virtually impossible during hypothermia, and diagnosis of brain dysfunction due to low perfusion pressure and low flow becomes difficult in a clinical setting where EEG may be the only diagnostic modality available. Recent studies by Govier et al. show that regional cerebral blood flow can be measured with the use of xenon 133 [15]. However, the technique requires sophisticated equipment and is unlikely to be available in most operating rooms. Because of the lack of a clinically useful cerebral function monitor in this situation, it becomes imperative that we maintain a safe perfusion pressure for brain protection.

Studies which show that low perfusion pressure and low flow maintain adequate cerebral autoregulation have been performed under stable hypothermic conditions and in normotensive patients with normal organ function. In reality, however, many of our patients have associated hypertension, carotid artery disease, renal dysfunction, and peripheral vascular disease. We have no evidence to suggest that, in these groups of patients, low pressure and low flow can be safely recommended. A steady state of hypothermia is maintained for a relatively short time in clinical practice. This is because patients are either being warmed or cooled for several minutes during CPB, and it may be more appropriate to maintain high perfusion pressures and flows during these times. Central nervous system dysfunction following open-heart surgery is a well-known phenomenon especially in the geriatric population [7, 16]. The spectrum of abnormalities varies from such mild symptoms as acute behavioral changes (mild cognitive dysfunction) to a much more serious diffuse or focal neurologic deficit [16, 18].

Although neurologic complications are common after all types of surgery, open-heart surgery poses added risks that can be attributed to CPB. In a study involving 35 patients undergoing open-heart surgery, Gilman showed that immediate postoperative neurologic abnormalities occurred in ~34% of patients [17]. Javid et al. (table 5-1) evaluated the incidence, the magnitude, and the reversibility of central nervous system disorders in 100 patients undergoing open-heart surgery [18]. Their study concluded that mean arterial pressure, age, and duration of CPB seemed to be the three most important factors contributing significantly to neurologic damage. In this study, the mean age of patients who demonstrated postoperative neurologic dysfunction and who

Table 5-1. Cerebral damage and blood pressure during bypass

Lowest level of mean arterial pressure recorded (mmHg)	Cerebral damage		Incidence per 100 patients
	Absent	Present	
≥60	8	3	27
50–59	18	15	45
40–49	17	21	55
≤40	4	14	78

subsequently survived was found to be 50.1 years, whereas that of patients with normal neurologic findings was only 43.4 years. These data suggest that older patients are more likely to develop neurologic complications. The authors also showed that mean arterial pressure below 50 mmHg was poorly tolerated when this was sustained for a prolonged period of time. The incidence of neurologic complications increased from 34% to 60% when the mean arterial pressure dropped below this critical level. Older patients seem to show a decreased tolerance for hypotension below 60 mmHg. Although the exact etiology of neurologic dysfunction occurring in patients undergoing CPB cannot always be determined with certainty, air and particulate emboli are major causes of this complication. Again, it is difficult to establish low flow and low arterial pressure as being the sole incriminating factors in neurologic deficit in any given situation.

In a study of 204 patients undergoing cardiac procedures, Slogoff et al. demonstrated that perfusion pressure, per se, was not the major determinent of postoperative neurologic dysfunction [7]. Other studies performed on similar patients essentially confirmed these findings in patients undergoing open-heart surgery. However, patients in these studies were all considered neurologically normal prior to the operation.

Postmortem examination of patients who demonstrated neurologic injury prior to death has revealed the presence of diffuse bilateral changes in the hippocampus [16]. Symmetric distribution of these lesions seems to be similar to the changes observed following episodes of ischemia. Although the presence of these lesions does not preclude microembolic etiology, the predominant hippocampal distribution is very suggestive of hypoxia as a result of hypoperfusion as the major causative factor.

It is well known that hypotension below a mean pressure of 50 mmHg is a common occurrence upon commencement of CPB as well as during rewarming. There is reason to believe that these two periods may be critical in the maintenance of adequate blood flow to the various tissues. In a study involving 29 adult patients undergoing cardiac surgery under enflurane anesthesia, Henriksen et al., using xenon 133, showed that blood flow decreased significantly in one patient who had a mean arterial blood pressure below 55 mmHg (figure 5-2) in the early stages of CPB [19]. A possible explanation for this

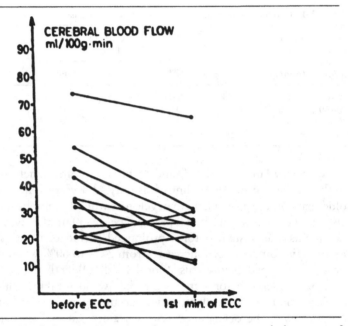

Figure 5-2. Cerebral blood flow in 12 patients between sternotomy and the onset of extracorporeal circulation (*ECC*), and in the initial phase (1st min) of *ECC*. In a patient with no flow in the second measurement, arterial pressure fell from 101 to 41 mmHg (Hendrickson et al).

phenomenon may lie in the fact that there is a release of catecholamines in the early stages of CPB, which can cause a shift of the cerebral autoregulation curve to the right, resulting in a diminished cerebral oxygen delivery at low perfusion pressures [20]. In these situations, there are no data to indicate that low perfusion pressure is safe for patients with hypertension and carotid artery disease. It would seem important that, in patients with hypertension and established cerebrovascular disease where flow is pressure dependent, perfusion pressure be maintained at a higher level than in normotensive patients. The incidence of stroke following CPB is 2%–5% [21, 22]. In patients with carotid artery disease, the incidence of stroke is related to the severity of stenosis and clinical manifestations. Although there is no definite evidence to show that patients do better postoperatively with higher perfusion pressures. Ivey et al. recommend that mean arterial pressure be maintained above 70 mmHg during CPB in patients with carotid artery stenosis measuring more than 50% of the diameter of the arterial lumen [23]. There were no focal neurologic events in patients that they studied in whom perfusion pressure was maintained at this level. However, the study was not supported by a control group for comparison.

Controversy still exists over the clinical significance of stump pressures measured on the ipsilateral side distal to the carotid stenosis. Hays et al., in a study of 197 patients, found that low carotid back pressure correlated well with the incidence of neurologic injuries [24]. Stockard et al., in a study involving 25 consecutive patients undergoing cardiac surgery, demonstrated that cerebral ischemia during CPB occurred in a pressure-dependent manner [25]. In their study, they developed a concept of *torr minutes* described as perfusion pressure below 50 torr (tm 50), a value represented geometrically by the area between the 50 torr line on the blood pressure record and the mean arterial pressure tracing when it was below 50 torr. For example, 100 tm 50 was equivalent to a 20-min period of perfusion pressure at 45 torr (20 × 5). They found that six (85.7%) of seven patients with hypotension index of greater than tm 50 manifested generalized neurologic deficits. Compared to this, only three (18.8%) of 16 with a hypotension index of less than 10 tm 50 had postoperative neurologic deficits. This study was conducted under moderate hypothermia (28°–32°C) and CPB was performed using a roller pump with a bubble oxygenator. Perfusion flows were maintained above 2.2 L/min/m² throughout CPB. The study underscores the importance of maintenance of a minimum perfusion pressure of 50 mmHg in patients undergoing cardiac surgery.

HYPERTENSION AND ADEQUACY OF CEREBRAL BLOOD FLOW (CBF)

CBF is known to be influenced by Pco_2, Po_2, body temperature, mean arterial pressure, intracranial pressure, and cerebral vascular resistance. Under awake, resting, normotensive, normocapnic conditions, changes in CBF are minimal. Autoregulation is an intrinsic protective mechanism whereby CBF remains constant over a wide range of cerebral perfusion pressure (CPP); the normal range of autoregulation varies between mean arterial pressures of 50 and 150 mmHg [26], which signifies that, when mean arterial pressure is less than 50 mmHg. CBF falls and the cerebral AVo_2 difference increases markedly, resulting in cerebral ischemia. On the other hand, when mean arterial pressure is above 150 torr, CBF increases steeply. Various factors such as ischemia, increase in Pco_2, vasodilator therapy, and acidosis will abolish the autoregulatory response and make brain perfusion pressure dependent [26–28].

In patients with chronic arterial hypertension, both upper and lower limits of the autoregulatory curve are shifted to the right [26–28]. This means that adequate oxygen delivery to the brain occurs at higher blood pressures (figure 5-3). Conversely, there may be cerebral ischemia when perfusion pressure drops to normotensive levels in patients who have chronic hypertension. Although the autoregulatory mechanism is reset at a higher level in these patients, controversy still exists as to the maximum drop in blood pressure that can be safely tolerated. Strandgaard et al. studied ten hypertensive patients and compared them to three normotensive patients as controls to demonstrate the effects of hypertension on cerebral function [29]. Ten hypotensive patients with blood pressures ranging from 160/100 to 250/145 mmHg were compared

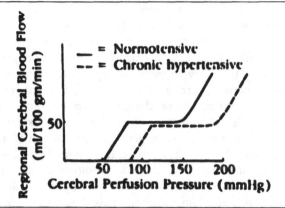

Figure 5-3. Cerebral autoregulation in both normotensive and chronic hypertensive patients whose actual limits of cerebral perfusion pressure depend on the degree of hypertension. Note the rightward shift of the hypertensive autoregulation curve.

with normotensive patients; in the hypertensive patients, the average mean blood pressure was 125 mmHg and that of normotensive patients was 70 mmHg. In the hypertensive group, the lowest mean blood pressure at which brain hypoxia occurred, as measured by AVo_2 difference, was 68 mmHg. CBF at this pressure was 73% of the resting level, Pco_2 being maintained at 35.8 mmHg. The lowest blood pressure at which brain hypoxia was seen to occur in the normotensive patients was 40 mmHg. CBF at this pressure was 66% of the resting level, Pco_2 being maintained at 34.5 mmHg. In three of ten hypertensive patients, AVo_2 difference decreased when the mean arterial pressure was raised above 160 mmHg, with an increase in CBF ranging from 17% to 60%. The normotensive patients demonstrated a 39% decrease in CBF when mean arterial pressure was raised above 120 mmHg. This study demonstrated that the lower limit of autoregulation in hypertensive patients was 120 mmHg, whereas in normotensive patients it was 70 mmHg.

It is clear that the perfusion pressure required to oxygenate the cerebral tissue of hypertensive patients adequately is considerably higher than that of normotensive patients, the hypothesis being that the rightward shift of autoregulation in hypertensive patients is possibly the result of hypertrophy of the arterial walls. This study not only emphasizes the importance of maintaining high perfusion pressures, but also explains why hypertensive patients are less likely to tolerate sudden hypotensive episodes. This also suggests that reduction in blood pressure of hypertensive patients should be undertaken gradually over a period of 1–2 months to allow time for the autoregulatory curve to shift back to the original position. There is also some evidence to show that a similar rightward shift of the autoregulatory curve occurs with increase in sympathetic activity of the nervous system. As such, during hypotensive periods on CPB, the use of vasoconstrictor drugs to increase mean arterial pressure is controver-

sial. This information is useful in realizing that patients can tolerate pharmacologically induced hypotension better than drops in blood pressure resulting
from hypovolemia because the latter is associated with increase in sympathetic
activity [26, 28]. In hypertensive patients, a decrease in mean arterial pressure
can be safely tolerated provided it does not exceed 50 mmHg from baseline
values, and provided the patients do not have a prior history of cerebrovascular disease or transient ischemic attacks [28]. These findings are
particularly relevant in patients undergoing cardiac surgery for aortocoronary
bypass because, in addition to a high incidence of associated hypertension,
they may also have artherosclerosis, which limits perfusion to vital organs. It
would probably be safe to recommend a higher perfusion pressure in these
patients. Farhat and Schneider have reported four cases illustrating the effect of
systemic hypertension and its role in cerebrovascular insufficiency [30]. They
concluded that the minimum, safe perfusion pressure is set at a higher level in
patients with hypertension with concomitant cerebrovascular insufficiency.

THE ROLE OF PERFUSION PRESSURE IN THE
MAINTENANCE OF CORONARY CIRCULATION

Myocardial ischemia or infarction can occur after aortocoronary bypass surgery. Depending on the criteria used for diagnosing ischemia, the reported
incidence is between 6% and 50% [31], the subendocardial region being the
most vulnerable anatomic area. It has been shown that the subendocardial
region is vulnerable to ischemia during normothermic arrest and induced
ventricular fibrillation [32, 33]. In hypertrophied ventricles and during
spontaneous fibrillation, the subendocardial zone is likely to become ischemic
at low perfusion pressures [34]. Although hypothermia reduces myocardial
oxygen consumption over time, the beat-to-beat oxygen consumption increases as a result of an increased inotropic state of the heart [35–37]. During
hypothermia, increase in MVO_2 is not associated with a concomitant increase
in the oxygen delivery. Oxygen delivery diminishes in these cases due to
increased contractile state of the ventricle and coronary vasoconstriction in
response to hypothermia [37, 38]. Additionally, Archie and Kirklin have
shown that the coronary vasodilator reserve capacity is reduced during hypothermia [36]. Increase in coronary vascular resistance is a result of increased
blood viscosity, increased vascular tone, and increased extravascular compression imposed by ventricular contractility.

When the coronary vasodilator reserve capacity decreases, flow distal to the
stenotic area becomes pressure dependent [39]. As a result, at low perfusion
pressure, the myocardium is vulnerable to ischemia. Therefore, hypothermia
does not provide protection against ischemia in the beating, empty heart at
perfusion pressures below 50 mmHg even though oxygen demand per unit
time is diminished. Fibrillating hypertrophic hearts may show an added propensity to subendocardial ischemia where hypothermia seems to be particularly
harmful.

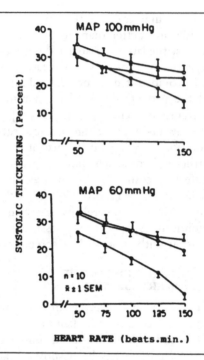

Figure 5-4. The effect of increase in heart rate and decrease in arterial blood pressure on systolic thickening of heart muscle. (C.W. Buffington).

Among the important factors influencing myocardial supply–demand ratio are heart rate and mean arterial pressure. In order to delineate the role of mean arterial pressure in the genesis of ischemia, Buffington has developed a dog model that has helped us better understand the effects of varying mean arterial pressure on myocardial ischemia in the presence of coronary stenosis [40]. Myocardial contractility was measured by implanting piezoelectric crystals in the epicardial and endocardial regions of the heart. Systolic thickening of the ventricle was used as an index of myocardial ischemia. The mean arterial pressure (MAP) was increased from 60 to 100 mmHg in four stages and, at each stage, the heart rate was increased from 50 to 150 beats/min in five segments. Systolic thickening was greatly diminished when mean blood pressure was decreased below 60 mmHg especially in combination with tachycardia (figure 5-4). Although this study was performed in the laboratory setting, the findings are relevant to CPB in that they clearly demonstrate the presence of ischemic myocardial dysfunction with reduction in mean perfusion pressure to below 60 mmHg.

Khuri et al. have emphasized the importance of perfusion pressure on CPB in patients with coronary artery disease [41]. In a canine study, they demonstrated convincingly that, in subjects with normal coronary arteries at MAP between 55 and 95 mmHg and flow rate of 50 ml/kg/min, there was no sign of myocardial ischemia. However, when subjected to MAP between 40 and 50 mmHg and flow rate 30 cc/kg/min, the animals became ischemic. When the MAP was increased to between 70 and 86 mmHg by clamping the decending aorta, these ischemic changes were abolished. After initiation of CPB at a flow rate of 41 ml/kg/min, the mean prebypass aortic pressure dropped from 107 to 49 mmHg and the circumflex coronary artery, which had previously been subjected to critical stenosis, showed a drop in flow from 27 to 13 ml/min. As a result, posterior wall myocardial CO_2 tension rose from 70 to 177 mmHg, indicating severe ischemia. When the mean aortic pressure was increased to 112 mmHg from 49 mmHg by clamping the aorta, there was an increase in circumflex coronary artery flow from 13 ml to 34 ml/min. There was a concomitant reduction in myocardial CO_2 tension to 74 mmHg, demonstrating clearly that a decrease in perfusion pressure in a critically constricted coronary vessel produced significant ischemia that could be corrected by elevating the MAP to prebypass levels (figure 5-5).

McConnell et al. have attempted to show the effect of perfusion pressure on hypothermia in the beating, nonworking heart during CPB with regard to myocardial blood flow and metabolism [39]. The study was conducted in dogs during normothermia at 37°C and hypothermia at 28°C, perfusion pressures being maintained at 100 and 50 mmHg. When the perfusion pressure was decreased from 100 to 50 mmHg, coronary sinus O_2 content decreased and there was a hyperemic response upon release of the coronary obstruction. Coronary flow decreased by 58% when perfusion pressure was reduced to 50 mmHg. It was shown that during normothermia, when perfusion pressure fell from 100 to 50 mmHg, blood flow to the left ventricle decreased with no change in the endocardial–epicardial flow ratio. However, during hypothermia, with a similar drop in blood pressure, the subendocardial flow decreased significantly more than flow to other regions of the myocardium. This study seems to indicate that, whereas the total blood flow to the myocardium is diminished with a decrease in perfusion pressure during normothermia, normal distribution of blood to various organs of the myocardium is maintained. During hypothermia, the distribution of blood is deviated away from the subendocardial region, making this zone more vulnerable to ischemic changes (figure 5-6). Decrease in perfusion pressure did not significantly alter myocardial oxygen consumption. However, there was a 20% drop in oxygen uptake when the perfusion pressure fell below 50 mmHg, signifying that oxygen delivery was impaired. During hypothermia, the left ventricle extracted 46% of the oxygen delivered when the perfusion pressure was maintained above 100 mmHg, and there was a slight rise in oxygen extraction when the pressure was reduced to 50 mmHg. This can be explained by the fact that the coronary blood flow was reduced by 60% at low pressures, again emphasizing the advantage of higher pressures (figure 5-7).

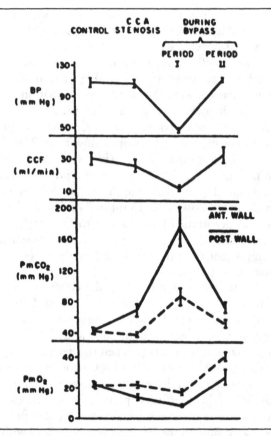

Figure 5-5. Changes in blood pressure (*BP*), circumflex coronary artery flow (*CCF*), and myocardial gas tension (*CMo₂*) in group 3 animals. Mean values ± SE; *CCA*, circumflex coronary artery.

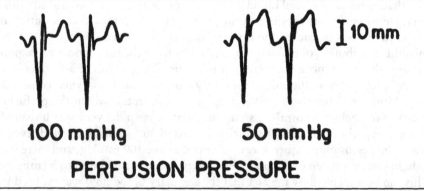

Figure 5-6. Intracavitary electrocardiogram during hypothermia (28°C). Note the elevation in the ST segments when perfusion pressure is lowered from 100 to 50 mmHg. (Khuri et al.).

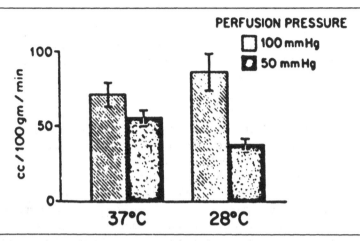

Figure 5-7. Left ventricular subendocardial blood flow of beating, nonworking heart at 37°C and 28°C with perfusion pressures at 100 and 50 mmHg. Note (a) the relative maintenance of subendocardial flow when perfusion pressure is reduced to 50 mmHg at 37°C, and (b) the fall in subendocardial flow when perfusion pressure is lowered during hypothermia (28°C), (McConnell et al.).

GASTROINTESTINAL COMPLICATIONS AND CPB

The incidence of gastrointestinal complications after CPB is reported to be 0.85%–1.0% [42]. These complications which include pancreatitis, cholecystitis, hyperbilirubinemia, and ischemic bowel syndrome, are associated with high morbidity and mortality. The incidence of increased serum amylase after CPB is reported to be as high as 30%, but clinical pancreatitis is quite rare. The incidence of pancreatitis as diagnosed by necropsy examination has been reported to be 3%–16% by various authors [5, 43–45]. Low cardiac output states were incriminated as a cause of ischemic bowel syndrome [46]. In this regard, since ischemic bowel is observed more frequently in patients who display myocardial pump failure, it is difficult to establish low perfusion pressure during CPB as the etiologic factor.

RENAL DYSFUNCTION AND CPB

Renal failure after coronary artery bypass surgery often carries a grave prognosis. In patients with renal failure, mortality ranges from 35% to 88%, depending on the severity of the disease [47–49]. Several studies indicate that preoperative left ventricular function, prolonged CPB, prolonged aortic cross-clamp time are major etiologic factors [47, 49, 50]. Senning et al., in a canine study, have demonstrated that the CPB decreases renal function as a result of decreased renal blood flow and decreased glomerular filtration rate, resulting in diminished electrolyte excretion [51]. These findings are more pronounced when low perfusion pressure and low flow are utilized on CPB. Yeboah et al.

have shown that mean arterial pressure above 80 mmHg significantly decreased the incidence of postoperative renal failure [47]. Connors has suggested that chronic renal failure patients be maintained at a flow rate of 2.4 L/min/m² during CPB, but the reasons for these recommendations are not clearly stated in his study [52].

CONCLUSION

In this chapter, we have attempted to highlight the role of high perfusion pressure and flow on CPB. There is recent evidence to show that low pressure and flow states can be safely tolerated under well-controlled hypothermic conditions in patients undergoing cardiac surgery without associated diseases. However, in a subgroup of patients demonstrating hypertension, central nervous system dysfunction, carotid occlusive disease, coronary artery disease, renal dysfunction, and generalized artherosclerotic disease, low pressure and low flow may be detrimental to organ perfusion. In addition to this, patients on CPB have diminished oxygen–carrying capacity due to anemia and iatrogenic respiratory alkalosis; also, uniform body cooling is not always achieved. In these situations, the efficacy and safety or low perfusion pressure have not been adequately established. Until we have more data to show that low perfusion pressure can be well tolerated in these situations. the current recommendation would be to maintain these patients at perfusion pressures higher than 50 mmHg and flow rates in excess of 1.5 L/min/m².

REFERENCES

1. Buckberg GD, Towers B, Paglia DE, Mulder DG, Maloney JV: Subendocardial ischemia after cardiopulmonary bypass. J Thorac Cardiovasc Surg 66:754, 1973.
2. Rose MR, Glassman E, Isom OW, Spencer FC: Electrocardiographic and serum enzyme changes of myocardial infarction after coronary artery bypass surgery. Am J Cardiol 33:215, 1974.
3. Kolkka R, Hilberman M: Neurologic dysfunction following cardiac operation with low flow, low pressure cardiopulmonary bypass. J Thorac Cardiovasc Surg 79:432–437, 1980.
4. Hiberman M, Myers BD, Carrie BJ: Acute renal failure following cardiac surgery. J Thorac Cardiovasc Surg 79:432–437, 1980.
5. Rose DM, Ranson JHC, Cunningham JN, Spencer FC: Patterns of severe pancreatic injury following cardiopulmonary bypass. Ann Surg 199: , 1984.
6. Robertson R, Dodds WA: Mesenteric artery insufficiency complicating repair of aortic regurgitation. Can J Surg 7:269–276, 1964.
7. Slogoff S, Girgis KZ, Ketas AS: Etiologic factors in neuropsychiatric complications associated with cardiopulmonary bypass. Anesth Analg 61:903–911, 1982.
8. Guyton AC: Transport of oxygen and carbon dioxide in the blood and body fluids. In: Textbook of medical phsyiology, 6th edn. WB Saunders, pp 504–515.
9. Linton RAP: Pulmonary gas exchange and acid base status. In: Churchill-Davidson HC (ed) A practice of anesthesia. Lloyd-Luke, pp 89–124.
10. Millar RD, Brzica SM: Blood components, colloids and autotransfusion therapy. In: Millar RD (ed) Anesthesia, vol. 2, 2nd edn. Churchill Livingstone, 1329–1367.
11. Kawashima I, Yamamoto Z. Manabe H: Safe limits of hemodilution in cardiopulmonary bypass. Surgery 76:391–397, 1974.
12. Litwak RS, Gadboys HL, Kahn M, Wisoff G: High flow total body perfusion utilizing diluted perfusate in a large prime system. J Thorac Cardiovasc Surg 49:74–90, 1965.
13. Dennis RC, Hechtman HB, Berger RL. Vito L, Weiser RD, Valeri CR: Transfusion of 2, 3-

DPG enriched red blood cells to improve cardiac function. Ann Thorac Surg 26:17, 1978.

14. Moores WY: Oxygen delivery during cardiopulmonary bypass. In: Utley J (ed) Pathophysiology and techniques of cardiopulmonary bypass. Williams and Wilkins.

15. Govier AV, Reeves JG, McKay RD. et al.: Factors and their influence on regional cerebral blood flow during non-pulsatile cardiopulmonary bypass. Ann Thorac Surg 38:592–600, 1984.

16. Tufo HM, Ostfeld AM, Shekella R: Central nervous system dysfunction following open heart surgery. JAMA 212:1333–1340, 1970.

17. Gilman S: Cerebral disorders after open heart operations. N Engl J Med 272:489–498, 1965.

18. Javid H, Tufo HM, Najafi H, Dve WS, Hunter JA, Julian OC: Neurological abnormalities following open heart surgery. J Thorac Cardiovasc Surg 58:502–509, 1969.

19. Henriksen L, Hjelms E, Lindeburgh T: Brain hyperfusion during cardiac operations. J Thorac Cardiovasc Surg 86:202–208, 1983.

20. Fitch W, Mackenzie ET, Harper AM: Effects of decreasing arterial pressure in cerebral blood flow in baboon: influence of sympathetic nervous system. Circ Res 37:550–567, 1975.

21. Breslau PJ, Fell G, Ivey TD, Bailey WW, Millar DW, Strandness DE: Carotid arterial disease in patients undergoing coronary artery bypass operations. J Thorac Cardiovasc Surg 82:765–767, 1981.

22. Reul GH, Morris GC, Howell JF, et al.: Current concepts in coronary artery surgery. Ann Thorac Surg 14:243–259, 1972.

23. Ivey TD, Strandness E, Williams DB, Langlois Y, Misbach GA, Kruse AP: Management of patients with carotid bruit undergoing cardiopulmonary bypass. J Thorac Cardiovasc Surg 87:183–189, 1984.

24. Hays RJ, Levinson SA, Wylie EJ: Intraoperative measurement of carotid back pressure as a guide to operative management of carotid endarterectomy. Surgery 72:953–960, 1973.

25. Stockard JJ, Bickford RB, Schauble JF: Pressure dependent cerebral ischemia during cardiopulmonary bypass. Neurology 23:521–529, 1973.

26. Lassen NA: Cerebral and spinal cord blood flow. In: Cottrell JE, Turndorf H (eds) Anesthesia and neurosurgery. CV Mosby, pp 1–24.

27. Donegan J: Physiology and metabolism of brain and spinal cord. In: Neufield P, Cotrell J (eds) Handbook of neuroanesthesia. Little, Brown and Company, Boston pp 2–15.

28. Shapiro HM: Anesthesia effects upon cerebral blood flow, cerebral metabolism, EEG and evoked potential. In: Millar RD (ed) Anesthesia, vol 2, 2nd edn. Churchill Livingstone, pp 1249–1288.

29. Strandgaard S. Olesen J, Skinhoj E, Larsen NA: Autoregulation of brain circulation in severe arterial hypertension. Br Med J 1:507–510, 1973.

30. Farhat SM, Schneider RC: Observations on the effect of systemic blood pressure on intracranial circulation in patients with cerebrovascular insufficiency. J Neurosurg 1967.

31. Engelman RM, Spencer FC, Boyd AD, Chandra R: The significance of coronary arterial stenosis during cardiopulmonary bypass. J Thorac Cardiovasc Surg 70:869–879, 1975.

32. Stemmer E, McCart P, Stanton W, Thibault W, Dearden L, Connolly JE: Functional and structural alterations in the myocardium during aortic cross clamping. J Thorac Cardiovasc Surg 66:754, 1973.

33. Hottenrott C, Towers B, Kurkji HJ, Maloney JV, Buckerg G: The hazard of ventricular fibrillation in hypertrophied ventricles during cardiopulmonary bypass. J Thorac Cardiovasc Surg 66:742–752, 1973.

34. Hottenrott C, Maloney JV, Buckberg G:Studies of the effects of ventricular fibrillation on the adequacy of regional myocardial flow mechanism of ischemia. J Thorac Cardiovasc Surg 68:634–645, 1974.

35. Goldberg LI: Effects of hypothermia on contractility of the infarct dog heart. Am J Physiol 194:9, 1958.

36. Archie JP, Kirklin JW: Effect of hypothermic perfusion on myocardial oxygen consumption and coronary resistance. Surg Forum 24:186, 1973.

37. Monroe RG, Strange RH, Lafarge CG, Levy J: Ventricular performance, pressure volume relationship and O_2 consumption during hypothermia. Am J Physiol 206:67, 1964.

38. Penrod KE: Cardiac oxygenation during severe hypothermia in dogs. Am J Physiol 164:79, 1951.

39. McConnell DH, Brazier JR, Cooper N, Buckberg GD: Studies of the effects of hypothermia on regional myocardial blood flow and metabolism during cardiopulmonary bypass. J Thorac

Cardiovasc Surg 73:95–101, 1977.
40. Buffington CW: Hemodynamic determinants of ischemic myocardial dysfunction in the presence of coronary stenosis in dogs. Anesthesiology 63:651–662, 1985.
41. Khuri SF, Brawley RK, O'Riordan JB, Donahoo JS, Pitt B, Gott VL: The effect of cardiopulmonary bypass perfusion pressure on myocardial gas tensions in the presence of coronary stenosis. Ann Thorac Surg 20:661–670, 1975.
42. Hanks JB, Curtis SE, Hanks BB, Anderson DK, Cox JL, Jones RS: Gastrointestinal complications after cardiopulmonary bypass. Surgery 92:394–400, 1982.
43. Panebianco AC, Scott SM, Dart CH. Takaro T, Echegaray HM: Acute pancreatitis following extracorporeal circulation. Ann Thorac Surg 9:562–568, 1970.
44. Feiner H: Pancreatitis after cardiac Surg. Am J Surg 684:131–135, 1976.
45. Warshaw AL, O'Hara PJ: Susceptibility of the pancreas to ischemic injury in shock. Ann Surg 188:197–220, 1978.
46. Horton EH, Murthy SK, Seal RME: Hemorrhagic necrosis of small intestine and acute pancreatitis following open heart surgery. Thorax 23:438–441, 1968.
47. Yeboah ED, Petrie A, Pead JL: Acute renal failure and open heart surgery. Br Med J 1:415–418. 1972.
48. Hilberman M, Myers BD, Carrie BJ, Derby G, Jamison RL, Stinson ED: Acute renal failure following cardiac surgery. 77:880–888, 1979.
49. Abel RM, Buckley MJ, Austen WG, Barnett GO, Beck CH Jr, Fischer JE: Etiology, incidence and prognosis of renal failure following cardiac operations. J Thorac Cardiovasc Surg 71:323–333, 1976.
50. Bhat JG, Gluck M, Lowenstein J, Baldwin DS: Renal failure after open heart surgery. Ann Intern Med 84:677–682, 1976.
51. Senning A, Andres J, Bornstein P, Norberg B, Nadersen MN: Renal function during extracorporeal circulation at high and low flow rates: experimental studies in dogs. Ann Surg 151:63–70, 1960.
52. Connors JP: Cardiopulmonary bypass in chronic renal disease. In: Utley (ed) Pathophysiology and techniques of cardiopulmonary bypass. Williams and Wilkins, pp 55–62.

6. LOW PRESSURE DURING CARDIOPULMONARY BYPASS IS PREFERABLE

J. G. REVES
ANN GOVIER
NARDA CROUGHWELL

Sustaining the circulation during cardiac operations requires use of extracorporeal circulation with a cardiopulmonary bypass (CPB) pump perfusion system. The safety of this procedure is remarkable when one ponders the technological, physiologic, and pathologic problems that have been encountered, solved, or ignored. [1] The perfusion pressure during CPB is one of the physiologic variables that usually becomes very abnormal, especially at the initiation of CPB. It is common for the perfusion pressure to decrease significantly to very low levels (20–30 mmHg) at the start of extracorporeal circulation. This degree of hypotension in normal man would certainly produce shock (inadequate tissue perfusion), but does not do so during the altered physiologic state of CPB. Nevertheless, there are valid reasons for concern when the perfusion pressure is diminished during CPB. We address these concerns as they apply to two organ systems: the brain and the heart.

"NORMAL" CARDIOPULMONARY BYPASS

The normal or customary conduct of CPB requires (a) a mechanical pump and oxygenator, (b) a pump prime designed to deliver a significantly reduced hematocrit (25–50% reduction), and (c) hypothermia. These three requirements are major departures from normal circulatory conditions. CPB per se is not innocuous and produces damaging effects [2] (figure 6-1). The damaging effects of CPB no doubt are the result of the abnormal physiologic conditions *and* the body's response to these conditions (e.g., release of catecholamines, prostaglandins, and complement).

99

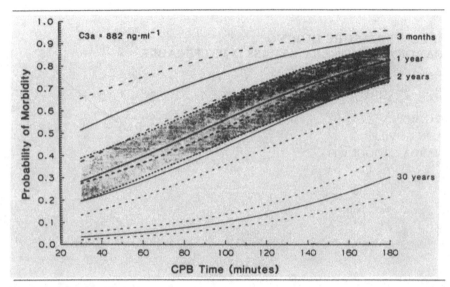

Figure 6-1. Nomogram from multivariate analysis (table 2-6) of the probability of morbidity (cardiac, pulmonary, renal, and coagulation dysfunction) after CPB. The presentation shows CPB time along the *horizontal axis*, and the relationships are shown for four age groups at a C3a level of 882 ng·ml^{-1} (the median value in the study). With permission, from Kirklin and Barratt-Boyes [1].

The perfusion pressure during nonpulsatile CPB may be described mathematically:

$$P_{SA} - P_{RA} = Q \times SVR \tag{1}$$

where P_{SA} is mean systemic pressure, P_{RA} is mean right atrial pressure, Q is flow, and SVR is systemic vascular resistance.

However, with proper gravity drainage, P_{RA} is zero and the equation becomes:

$$P_{SA} = Q \times SVR \tag{2}$$

During CPB, Q is manipulated by the perfusionists and is limited by the venous return to the pump and/or the flow capability of the pump (all pumps have maximal flow capacity). SVR is determined by two factors: the vascular resistance and the blood viscosity [3]. The relationship is:

$$SVR = \eta \times VR \tag{3}$$

where η is blood viscosity and VR is vascular resistance.

Substituting formulas 1, 2, and 3, we get an equation 4 useful in considering perfusion pressure during CPB:

$$P_{SA} = Q \times \eta \times VR \tag{4}$$

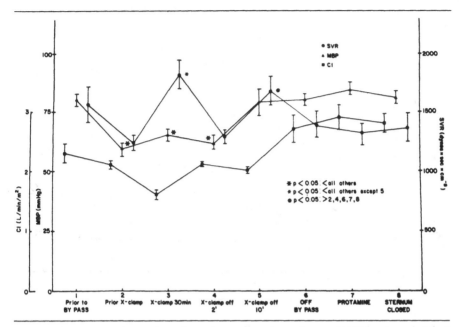

Figure 6-2. Mean cardiac index (*CI*), systemic vascular resistance (*SVR*), and mean blood pressure (*MBP*) during cardiac anesthesia and surgery. *Bars* indicate SEM. With permission, from Reves et al. [8].

Thus, the perfusion pressure during CPB is a product of the pump flow, the viscosity of the perfusate, and the vascular resistance.

The perfusion pressure decreases during CPB, especially at the initiation of CPB. The normal course of P_{SA} (MBP) as well as cardiac index (CI) and systemic vascular resistance during CPB is shown in figure 6-2. The SVR usually has its nadir at the onset of CPB, increases during the time of normal hypothermia and aortic cross-clamping, and again decreases with rewarming.

It is not our purpose to review in detail the multiple factors related to the changes in P_{SA} during CPB, but since $P_{SA} = Q \times \eta \times VR$, and it is known that Q does not change much during CPB (figure 6-2), then the reduction in P_{SA} must be due to decreases in viscosity and vascular resistance. The viscosity does indeed drop and the change in P_{SA} is reasonably well correlated ($r = 0.67$, $p < 0.01$) [4]. The change in viscosity is reflected by the degree of hemodilution (change in hematocrit). There are significant reductions in SVR [5–7] that affect P_{SA}, but the mechanisms are unknown. Rises in SVR during CPB parallel increases in plasma norepinephrine [8].

The use of hypothermic perfusion is important. The lowered temperature negates some of the effects of changes in viscosity since decreases in temperature will increase viscosity; however, the more important aspect of hypothermia is its effect on organ metabolism. As temperature is reduced, the

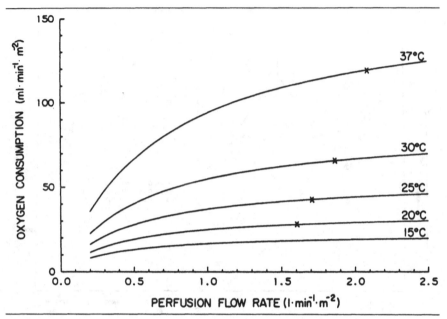

Figure 6-3. Nomogram of an equation expressing the relationship of oxygen consumption (V_2O_2) to perfusion flow rate (Q) and temperature (T). The small x's have been added to represent the perfusion flow rates used clinically at these temperatures. With permission, from Kirklin and Barratt-Boyes [1].

various organs have reduced metabolism and less oxygen utilization. Thus the oxygen consumption (V_{O_2}) of organs is reduced with hypothermic CPB. It is assumed that the reduction in metabolic rate for V_{O_2} protects tissue from relative oxygen deprivation that occurs at lowered perfusion flows and pressures. The relationship of decrease in V_{O_2} to temperature can be expressed as the Q_{10}, which means that a 10°C change in temperature is accompanied by a twofold change in V_{O_2} [1]. The Q_{10} for man on CPB is ~3: this means that a decrease in temperature of 10°C should reduce V_{O_2} at least 50%.

Temperature alone does not affect V_{O_2}. The flow (Q) will also alter V_{O_2}: in fact, there is a best-fit hyperbolic relationship between perfusion flow rate and V_{O_2} that occurs at lower flow. The interrelationship of temperature and flow to V_{O_2} is shown in figure 6-3. In this normogram, various flows and temperatures are plotted against V_{O_2} in an attempt to define *optimal* flow temperature conditions during CPB. It is apparent that normotheric flow should be 2.0 L/min/m² whereas at 25°C 1.6 L/min/m² is sufficient [1]. Thus, the clinical recommendations for appropriate flow are made to provide adequate oxygenation of tissues and depend on temperature of the patient during CPB. Lower flows are safe in hypothermic patients and, conversely, with rewarming, flow needs to be increased (to the low normal physiologic range).

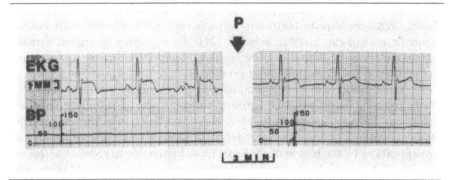

Figure 6-4. ECG (leds V$_5$) and systemic blood pressure (*BP*) in a 69-year-old woman with multivessel coronary artery disease. Note ST elevation at perfusion pressure of 45–50 mmHg that resolves 3 min after phenylephrine (*P*) and with elevation of BP to 75–80 mmHg. Flow was 5 liters/min (2.4 L/min/m^2), temperature 33°C, and hematocrit 22 vol%.

ADEQUACY OF MYOCARDIAL PERFUSION

Since the purpose of cardiac surgery is to preserve or improve cardiac function, it is obvious that procedures or techniques that damage the heart are undesirable [9]. The perfusion pressure decreases with initiation of CPB. Does this jeopardize myocardial perfusion and attempts to protect the heart from damage? There are remarkably few clinical studies addressing this important question. Figure 6-4 shows the electrocardiogram and systemic blood pressure in a patient with ischemic heart disease. With a perfusion pressure of 50 mmHg, ST evidence of ischemia occurred in lead V$_5$. After phenylephrine administration and restoration of the systemic pressure to 80 mmHg, the ST elevations were markedly decreased. Such a case suggests that low perfusion pressure may lead to myocardial ischemia prior to aortic cross-clamping despite the fact that the heart is cooled and not working during early CPB and should be protected from ischemia by virtue of reduced oxygen requirements. The incidence of ischemia during CPB prior to aortic cross-clamping is not known, but it is not always present even at very low perfusion pressure.

A number of very good laboratory studies have investigated the effect of perfusion pressure on global and regional myocardial blood flow during CPB. The conditions of these studies may be grouped according to some of the important physiologic experimental conditions of temperature, pressure, systemic flow, hemodilution, and presence of critical stenosis with and without collateral circulation. *Hemodilution* requires greater flow to the heart to maintain oxygen supply because, with hemodilution, oxygen-carrying capacity is reduced [10]. The use of *hypothermia* also has implications for adequacy of myocardial oxygenation. Although hypothermia reduces myocardial oxygen consumption, it alters the determinants of supply (O$_2$ content, O$_2$ release from hemoglobin, and coronary flow). Hypothermia shifts the oxhyhemoglobin dissociation curve (to the left), making it more difficult to release O_2 to the tissues. With inadequate perfusion, hypothermic (28°C) hearts with normal coronary arteries can become ischemic [11]. Thus, it may be argued that the customary clinical conditions of hemodilution and hypothermia are not protective if adequate perfusion is not preserved.

Other conditions can impair adequacy of coronary perfusion during CPB. These are *reduction of perfusion pressure*, the presence of significant *coronary obstruction*, and *ventricular hypertrophy*. The importance of perfusion pressure has been shown in a number of laboratory studies [11–14]. The subendocardium appears to be the region of the heart most vulnerable to reduced perfusion pressure. The empty beating heart is probably adequately perfused with pressure ≥60 mmHg [12], but there is a significant reduction in flow to the heart and especially subendocardium at systemic pressures less than 50 mmHg.

The presence of a stenotic lesion and low perfusion pressure has been shown to produce ischemia [13, 14]. In an early study of this problem, Khuri and co-workers demonstrated that, when a perfusion pressure of less than 40–60 mmHg occurred during CPB, myocardial O_2 decreased and that CO_2 increased (evidence of hypoxic ischemia) [14]. The ischemia could be reversed by elevating the perfusion pressure nonpharmacologically (by aortic constriction). Myocardial ischemia was more pronounced in areas where an acute coronary constriction was made. Thus, ischemia that is perfusion pressure dependent is worsened by the presence of a coronary obstruction, presumably the same as is clinically encountered in patients with coronary artery disease.

The question that still remains is whether there is appropriate therapy for hypotension-associated myocardial ischemia during CPB. It is well known that coronary arteries will constrict in response to α-1 stimulation [15, 16]. There is clear evidence that raising the perfusion pressure by α-1 agonists like phenylephrine [17] and methoxamine [18] will improve the global cardiac blood flow and better perfuse the subendocardium in animals with normal coronary arteries during CPB. However, in animals with chronic (1 month) coronary constriction and those with developed collateral flow, raising the perfusion pressure from 50 to 80 mmHg with phenylephrine compromises blood flow to the vulnerable endocardium supplied by constricted and collateral arteries [17] (figure 6-5). These data raise the very important clinical question of the benefit of treating hypotension with an α-1 agonist. It may be that those areas of the heart most likely to sustain ischemic damage due to hypotension may be actually further compromised by use of α-1 agonists. It probably is rational to increase the pump flow in an attempt to raise perfusion pressure, especially in cases where there is evidence of ischemia, but treatment with α-1 agonists may not be beneficial.

ADEQUACY OF CEREBRAL PERFUSION

Early studies indicated an increased incidence of cerebral complications in patients with low arterial pressures during CPB [19, 20]. Studies by Tufo

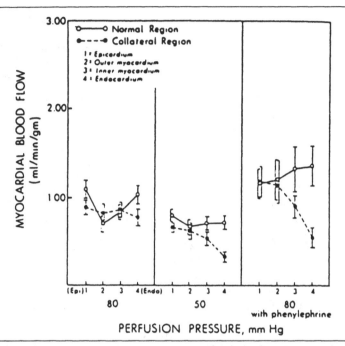

Figure 6-5. Transmural myocardial blood flow (ml/min/g) at the control 80 mmHg perfusion pressure, at 50 mmHg perfusion pressure, and at 80 mmHg perfusion pressure with phenylephrine infusion. The normal region is represented by the *solid lines* and the collateral region by *broken lines*. The epicardium (*Epi*) is represented as *layer 1* and the endocardium (*Endo*) as *layer 4*. Intermediate ventricular layers are shown as *numbers 2 and 3*. Note the distribution of blood flow away from the endocardium of the collateral region with phenylephrine infusion. With permission, from Sink et al. [17].

et al. [21] in 1970 and Stockard et al. [22] in 1973 concluded that mean arterial pressure had to be maintained at greater than 50 mmHg to avoid postoperative disorders of cerebral function, presumably due to inadequate cerebral blood flow (CBF). However, Kolkka and Hilberman [23], in a prospective study of 204 patients who underwent cardiac operations with hypothermic CPB, found no correlation of perfusion pressure with postoperative neurologic dysfunction. Their study suggested that perfusion pressure, per se, is not the major determinant nor a reliable predictor of postoperative cerebral dysfunction in an orderly operative procedure with adequate CPB flow. Slogoff et al. [24], in a prospective study of 204 patients, were also unable to confirm the relationship between postoperative cerebral dysfunction and perfusion pressures less than 50 mmHg during hypothermic CPB, Recently, Nussmeier et al. [25] confirmed this in a study of 89 valvular heart-diseased patients.

Govier et al. [26] in 1984 studied the factors that influence regional CBF during nonpulsatile hypothermic CPB. Regional CBF was determined by xenon-133 clearance in 67 patients undergoing coronary artery bypass graft

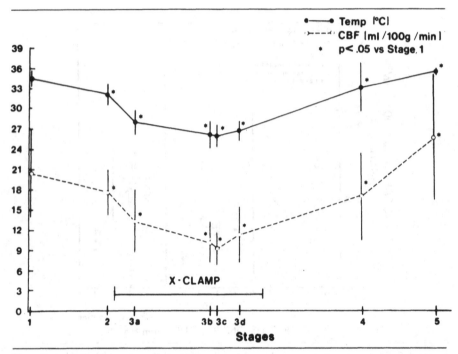

Figure 6-6. Cerebral blood flow (*CBF*) and nasopharyngeal temperature (*Temp*) during stages 1–5 of the surgical procedures. Note the parallel changes in temperature and CBF. *Stage 1*, 5–10 min before cardiopulmonary bypass; *stage 2*, 5–10 min after initiation of CPB; *stage 3a*, first injection of xenon during CPB with aortia cross-clamped; *stage 3b*, second injection during CPB with aorta cross-clamped; *stage 3c*, third injection during CPB with aorta cross-clamped; *stage 3d*, fourth injection during CPB with aorta cross-clamped; *stage 4*, during CPB after release of aortic cross clamp; and *stage 5*, CPB. Data are shown as mean ± standard deviation. With permission, from Govier et al. [26].

procedures. Patients with known cerebrovascular disease or with preoperative hypertension (diastolic blood pressure higher than 90 mmHg) were excluded from the study. There was a significant decrease in regional CBF (55%) during CPB with nasopharyngeal temperature and $Paco_2$ being the only significant factors influencing CBF. Figure 6-6 shows the parallel relationship of regional CBF and nasopharyngeal temperature during CPB. There is a highly significant correlation of regional CBF with temperature during CPB. The changes in regional CBF during CPB are directly related to changes in temperature and presumably therefore cerebral metabolism. The 55% reduction in regional flow is most likely related to the calculated 56% reduction in cerebral metabolic rate for oxygen expected with the average 8°C decrease in temperature during CPB, assuming the Q_{10} for human brain to be 2.8 during CPB [28].

There is a poor association between regional CBF and mean arterial pressure (MAP) (figure 6-7), a finding consistent with preserved autoregulation. In fact, during hypothermic CPB, the lower limit of autoregulation appears to

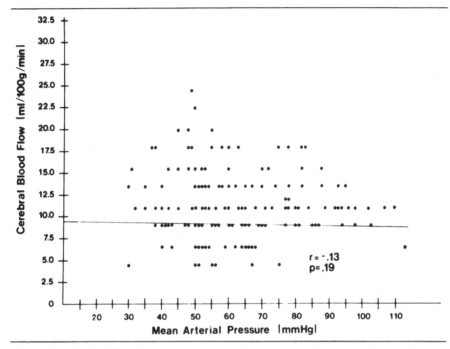

Figure 6-7. Cerebral blood flow versus mean arterial pressure during cardiopulmonary bypass. The *line* represents an average regression line over all patients. There are 44 hidden observations, i.e., data points, superimposed on each other. With permission, from Govier et al. [26].

be as low as 30 mmHg. This is in contrast to normotensive, normothermic human beings with a normal cerebrovascular status in whom autoregulation limits range between 50 and 150 mmHg. The most likely reason for the extension of the lower limit of autoregulation is that less CBF is required in the hypothermic state. Henriksen and associates [29] found that cerebral autoregulation was maintained down to arterial pressures of only ~55 mmHg. Below this level, they reported a significant association between regional CBF and MAP during CPB. The patients in that study received 1.5% enflurane as an anesthetic agent, which was discontinued at the time of CPB. Many anesthetic drugs interfere with cerebral autoregulation. The extent and duration of impairment of cerebral autoregulation due to enflurane are uncertain, but this is an important difference in anesthetic techniques between the two studies and may explain the discrepancy in the apparently lower limit of autoregulation.

Controversy exists regarding the optimal perfusion flow during hypothermic CPB. There are times when adequate surgical exposure may require very low rates of perfusion flow, and there is concern that the CBF may drop to inadequate levels during these periods of low perfusion flow. In all 67 patients, Govier et al. [26] found a marginally significant relationship of systemic blood flow (Q) to regional CBF (figure 6-8) and examined the influence of systemic

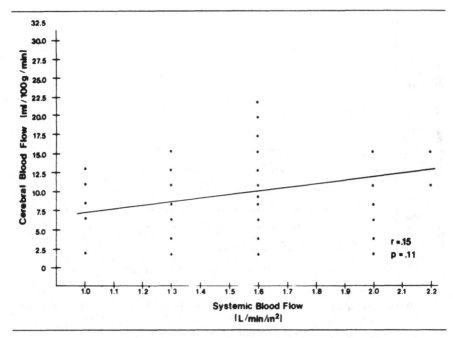

Figure 6-8. Cerebral blood flow versus systemic blood flow during cardiopulmonary bypass. The *line* represents an average regression line over all patients. With permission, from Govier et al. [26].

blood flow (Q) on regional CBF in ten patients by randomly varying flow and keeping MAP, nasopharyngeal temperature, and PA_{CO_2} relatively constant. The results indicate that there is no significant change in regional CBF measured during hypothermic CPB when Q is varied between 1.0 and 2.0 L/min/m² for short time intervals (minutes). Whole body oxygen consumption progressively falls as the rate of perfusion flow is decreased during hypothermic total CPB [30]; however, a study by Fox and associates [31] in cynomolgus monkeys revealed that brain oxygen consumption remained unchanged with decreasing perfusion flow rates. Apparently, tissue oxygenation is maintained in part by increased oxygen extraction and in part by redistribution of perfusate from the body to the brain. Cerebrovascular resistance remained unchanged at decreasing flow rates while the systemic circulation resistance increased. These findings partially corroborate findings by Govier et al. of a relatively constant regional CBF at varying perfusion flow rates in human beings, and is consistent with the hypothesis that cerebral autoregulation is preserved during cardiopulmonary bypass.

The minimental state exam (MMSE) is a test of cognitive function used by Freeman et al. [32] in 17 patients undergoing CPB in whom regional CBF was being measured by xenon 133. Freeman et al. did not find a relationship between postoperative cognitive dysfunction and age, duration of CPB, or lowered CBF during bypass. Their data reveal that low regional CBF encountered during hypothermic CPB does not contribute to clinical neurologic dysfunction or to subclinical dysfunction as tested by MMSE.

Importantly, it is now known that pharmacologic treatment of arterial pressures between 30 and 110 mmHg during hypothermic CPB is not necessary to insure constant cerebral blood flow in normotensive patients with normal cerebrovascular status. The previously held belief that the perfusion pressure should be maintained greater than 50 mmHg during CPB for cerebral protection cannot be defended solely on the premise that, below this level, CBF falls. In addition, the effects of the vasopressors on other organ systems, especially the heart (vide supra) and renal system, are not known in man during CPB and nonpulsatile flow. It is possible that the vasopressors may actually interfere with myocardial and renal perfusion to a greater degree than a lower perfusion pressure and further compromise these vital organs.

During CPB, just as in normothermic human beings, $Paco_2$ is an important factor modifying CBF. Increasing $Paco_2$ increases flow, while reduction in $Paco_2$ decreases flow. Patients in the study by Govier et al. were not exposed to hypercapnia, which may impair cerebral autoregulation [33]. They found a significantly direct correlation between regional CBF and $Paco_2$ during CPB, indicating that carbon dioxide tension is an important determinant of regional CBF during hypothermic CPB. Others [34, 35] have also found that carbon dioxide directly affects CBF during CPB. The optimal management and level of $Paco_2$ during hypothermic CPB have not been thoroughly studied. Recently Murkin (personal communication) demonstrated that the maintenance of temperature-corrected $Paco_2$ of 40 mmHg induced a profound cerebral hyperemia with significant uncoupling of oxygen supply from demand. This resulted in a disruption of cerebral autoregulation and produced pressure-passive CBF. It is not yet clear, however, whether there are upper and lower limits of $Paco_2$ beyond which the cerebral vessels do not react.

Unfortunately, there have been no studies performed on humans during hypothermic nonpulsatile CPB that assess the influence of significant carotid disease or cerebrovascular disease on CBF and autoregulation. Therefore, we cannot say with any certainty where the perfusion pressure should be maintained during CPB in these patients. However, recent data indicate that there is no relationship between incidence of perioperative strokes and the presence of high-grade carotid artery stenosis. Reports by Barnes et al. [36] and Turnipseed et al. [37] could not relate the incidence of perioperative strokes to the presence of high-grade carotid stenosis. Turnipseed et al. found no direct relationship between bruits, severity of disease, and the incidence of perioperative strokes. Of importance is that Turnipseed's study included patients with antecedent neurologic symptoms as well as patients that were asymptomatic. The data seem to indicate that, despite the presence of carotid stenosis, autoregulation may not be lost. It is known that, in normothermic, awake man, chronic hypertension shifts the entire autoregulation curve to the right [38].

As a result of this shift, the brain is better protected at high cerebral perfusion pressure, but may be more vulnerable to ischemia at low cerebral perfusion pressure. A variety of intracranial disorders may impair autoregulation. Additional studies are needed to address the impact of both cerebrovascular disease and hypertension on CBF during hypothermic CPB. If cerebral autoregulation is disturbed during bypass, regardless of the cause, it is possible that hypotension and associated decreased cerebral perfusion could produce central nervous system ischemic injury.

In summary, autoregulation of the CBF appears to exist in normotensive human beings during hypothermic CPB. The lower limit of cerebral autoregulation is extended to at least 30 mmHg during CPB at flow rates of 1.6 L/min/m^2 in moderately hypothermic patients. Due to autoregulation of CBF, it appears that pharmacologic support is not necessary to maintain a constant CBF between a MAP of 30 and 100 mmHg during CPB. With intact autoregulation, it appears that perfusion flow rates during hypothermic CPB may be reduced to as low as 1.0 L/min/m^2 for a short time interval without significantly reducing regional CPB. When more accurate, precise, noninvasive methods for measuring CBF in humans are developed, additional knowledge and understanding of the physiologic effect of CPB on man will hopefully decrease neurologic complications from cardiac operations.

CONCLUSION

Cardiopulmonary bypass is an abnormal physiologic state. Despite this, it is remarkably safe when used for reasonable time periods in relatively healthy patients. Treating a low perfusion pressure with α-1 agonist drugs has not been shown to affect outcome favorably. We therefore do not customarily treat hypotension other than by increasing pump flow to the range of 2.2–2.4 L/min/m^2. If there is persistent (>5–10 min) evidence of myocardial ischemia (such as ST changes), pharmacologic treatment is indicated. Other organ systems, like the renal, could suffer damage from hypotensive CPB during normal flow, but this has not been our experience. The cerebral circulation is preserved during CPB even at low perfusion pressures. Our recommendation is that hypotensive (30–50 mmHg) CPB conducted with hypothermia and normal flow (1.6–2.2 L/min/m^2) is well tolerated and is just one of the many abnormal physiologic conditions of extracorporeal perfusion. We do not routinely treat hypotension during hypothermic cardiopulmonary bypass.

ACKNOWLEDGMENTS

The authors wish to thank Ms. Laraine Goss for her expert clerical contributions to this work. A portion of this manuscript will appear in *Brain Dysfunction after Cardiac Surgery*, edited by Mark Hilberman and published by Martinus Nijhoff.

REFERENCES

1. Kirklin JW, Barratt-Boyes BG: *Cardiac surgery*. John Wiley and Sons, New York, 1986.
2. Kirklin JK, Westaby S, Blackstone EH, Kirklin JW, Chenoweth DE, Pacifico AD: Complement and the damaging effects of cardiopulmonary bypass. J Thorac Cardiovasc Surg 86:845–857, 1983.
3. Smith EE, Crowell JW: Role of an increased hematocrit in altitude acclimatization. Aerospace Med 38:39–443, 1967.
4. Gordon RJ, Ravin M, Daicoff GR, Rawitscher RE: Effects of hemodilution on hypotension during cardiopulmonary bypass. Anesth Analg Curr Res 54:482–488, 1975.
5. Wallach R, Karp RB, Reves JG, Oparil S, Smith LR, James TN: Pathogensis of paroxysmal hypertension developing during and after coronary bypass surgery: a study of hemodynamic and humoral factors. Am J Cardiol 46:559–565, 1980.
6. Reves JG, Buttner E, Karp RB, Oparil S, McDaniel HG, Smith LR: Elevated catecholamines during cardiac surgery: consequences of reperfusion of the postarrested heart. Am J Cardiol 53:722–728, 1984.
7. Cryer PE: Physiology and pathophysiology of the human sympathoadrenal neuroendo-crine system. N Engl J Med 303:436, 1980.
8. Reves JG, Karp RB, Buttner EE, Tosone S, Smith LR, Samuelson PN, Kreusch GR, Oparil S: Neuronal and adrenomedullary catecholamine release in response to cardiopulmonary bypass in man. Circulation 66:49–55, 1980.
9. Lell WA, Buttner E: Myocardial preservation during cardiopulmonary bypass. In: Kaplan J (ed) *Cardiac anesthesia, vol. 2: cardiovascular pharmacology*. Grune and Stratton, New York, 1983, pp 525–550.
10. Kleinman LH, Yarbrough JW, Symmonds JB, Wechsler AS: Pressure–flow characteristics of the coronary collateral circulation during cardiopulmonary bypass. J Thorac Cardiovasc Surg 75:17–27, 1978.
11. McConnell DH, Brazier JR, Cooper N, Buckberg GD: Studies of the effects of hypothermia on regional myocardial blood flow and metabolism during cardiopulmonary bypass. II. Ischemia during moderate hypothermia in continually perfused beating hearts. J Thorac Cardiovasc Surg 73:95–101, 1977.
12. Barid RJ, Dutka F, Okumori M, de la Rocha A, Goldbach MM, Hill JG, MacGregor DC: Surgical aspects of regional myocardial blood flow and myocardial pressure. J Thorac Cardiovasc Surg 69:17–29, 1975.
13. Engelman RM, Spencer FC, Boyd AD, Chandra R: The significance of coronary arterial stenosis during cardiopulmonary bypass. J Thorac Cardiovasc Surg 70:869–879, 1975.
14. Khuri SF, Brawley RK, O'Riordan JB, Donahoo JS, Pitt B, Gott VL: The effect of cardiopulmonary bypass perfusion pressure on myocardial gas tensions in the presence of coronary stenosis. Ann Thorac Surg 20:661–670, 1975.
15. Mohrman DE, Feigl EO: Competition between sympathetic vasoconstriction and metabolic vasodilation in the canine coronary circulation. Circ Res 42:79–86, 1978.
16. Vatner SF, Pagani M, Manders WT, Pasipoularides AD: Alpha adrenergic vasoconstriction and nitroglycerin vasodilation of large coronary arteries in the conscious dog. J Clin Invest 65:5–14, 1980.
17. Sink JD, Hill RC, Chitwood WR Jr, Abriss R, Wechsler AS: Effects of phenylephrine on transmural distribution of myocardial blood flow in regions supplied by normal and collateral arteries during cardiopulmonary bypass. J Thorac Cardiovasc Surg 78:236–243, 1979.
18. Symmonds JB, Kleinman LH, Wechsler AS: Effects of methoxamine on the coronary circulation during cardiopulmonary bypass. J Thorac Cardiovasc Surg 74:577–585, 1977.
19. Javid H, Tufo HM, Najafi H, Dys WS, Hunter JA, Julian OC: Neurological abnormalities following open heart surgery. J Thorac Cardiovasc Surg 58:502–509, 1969.
20. Branthwaite MA: Detection of neurological damage during open heart surgery. Thorax 28:464–72, 1973.
21. Tufo HM, Ostfeld AM, Shekelle R: Central nervous system dysfunction following open-heart surgery. JAMA 212:1333, 1970.
22. Stockard JJ, Bickford RG, Schauble JF: Pressure-dependent cerebral ischemia during cardio-pulmonary bypass. Neurology 23:521, 1973.

23. Kolkka R, Hilberman M: Neurologic dysfunction following cardiac operation with low flow, low pressure CPB. J Thorac Cardiovasc Surg 79:432, 1980.
24. Slogoff S, Girgis KZ, Keats AS: Etiologic factors in neuropsychiatric complications associated with CPB. Anesth Analg 61:903, 1982.
25. Nussmeier NA, Arlund C, Slogoff S: Neuropsychiatric complications after cardiopulmonary bypass: cerebral protection by a barbiturate. Anesthesiology 64:165–170, 1986.
26. Govier AV, Reeves JG, McKay RD, et al.: Factors and their influence on regional cerebral blood flow during nonpulsatile cardiopulmonary bypass. Am Thorac Surg 38:592, 1984.
27. Waltz AG, Wanek AR, Anderson RE: Comparison of analytic methods for calculation of cerebral blood flow after intracarotid injection of ^{133}Xe. J Nucl Med 13:66, 1972.
28. Kent B, peirce II EC: Oxygen consumption during cardiopulmonary bypass in the uniformly cooled dog. J Appl Physiol 37:917, 1974.
29. Henriksen L, Hjelms E, Lindeburgh T: Brain hyperperfusion during cardiac operations. J Thorac Cardiovasc Surg. 86:202, 1983.
30. Fox LS, Blackstone EH, Kirklin JW, et al.: Relationship of whole boyd oxygen consumption to perfusion flow rate during hypothermic cardiopulmonary bypass. J Thorac Cardiovasc Surg 83:239, 1982.
31. Fox LS, Blackstone EH, Kirklin JW, et al.: Relationship of brain blood flow and O_2 consumption to perfusion flow rate during profoundly hypothermic cardiopulmonary bypass: an experimental study. J Thorac Cardiovasc Surg 87:658, 1984.
32. Freeman AM, Folk DG, Sokol R, et al.: Cognitive function after coronary bypass surgery: effect of decreased cerebral blood flow. Am J Psychiatry 142:110, 1985.
33. Govier et al.
34. Wollman H, Stephen GW, Clement AJ, Danielson GK: Cerebral blood flow in man during extracorporeal circulation. J Thorac Cardiovasc Surg 52:558, 1966.
35. Kubota Y: Clinical study of the cerebral hemodynamics during extracorporeal circulation. Nagoya J Med Sci 13:117, 1968.
36. Barnes RW, Liebman PR, Marszalek PB, et al.: the natural history of asymptomatic carotid disease in patients undergoing cardiovascular surgery. Surgery 90:1075, 1981.
37. Turnipseed WD, Berkoff HA, Blezer FO: Postoperative stroke in cardiac and peripheral vascular disease. Ann Surg 192:365, 1980.
38. Michenfelder JG: The cerebral circulation. In: Prys-Roberts P (ed) The circulation in anaesthesia. Blackwell, Oxford, 1980, pp 209–225.

7. PULMONARY ARTERY CATHETERS SHOULD BE USED ROUTINELY IN ALL PATIENTS UNDERGOING CORONARY ARTERY BYPASS GRAFTING

MARTIN J. LONDON
DENNIS T. MANGANO

To "prove" that pulmonary artery (PA) catheters should be routinely employed in all patients undergoing coronary artery bypass graft surgery (CABG) surgery, we present the following four arguments and their rationales:

1. Based on the results of the major outcome trials comparing surgical to medical management in the treatment of coronary artery disease, patients now being referred for surgical therapy have a greater number of risk factors that may complicate their anesthetic management.
2. PA monitoring provides valuable hemodynamic data not obtainable by physical examination or central venous pressure (CVP) monitoring. Its use is essential to direct the safe conduct of perioperative anesthetic management.
3. CABG surgery is very expensive. The added cost of PA monitoring is insignificant when compared to the overall cost. Its use to guide more effective therapy can actually reduce overall cost.
4. PA monitoring has been shown to be a safe procedure. Its complications can be minimized by a thorough knowledge of the procedure along with careful attention to detail.

ARGUMENT 1

Risk profiles of patients presenting for CABG surgery have been radically redefined by the results of the three major randomized clinical trials of outcome comparing CABG surgery to medical therapy (Coronary Artery Surgery

Study [CASS], European Coronary Surgery Study [ECSS], and the Veterans Administration Cooperative Study [VA]). The widespread acceptance of per-cutaneous transluminal coronary angioplasty (PTCA) as an alternate to CABG surgery has also had significant impact. Patients now presenting for surgery are "sicker", with moderate-to-severe impairment of ventricular function, advanced degrees of coronary artery disease, older age, concurrent medical illnesses, and may have undergone previous CABG surgery.

CABG surgery has been aptly described by Pluth [1] as "the most expensive medical therapy applicable to the greatest number of patients in the history of mankind." The overall cost of the operation ranges from $15,000 to $25,000 per patient [2–4]. The number of procedures performed in this country has grown from 20,000 in 1971 to 191,000 in 1983. Given these numbers, the pro-cedure was estimated to account for ~1% of the nation's annual health care cost in 1980 [2]. Lenfant and Roth [2], using Lewis Thomas' definitions of the three levels of the *technology of medicine*, classify CABG surgery as an example of *halfway technology*, representing that which must be done to compensate for the incapacitating effects of disease or to postpone death. They indicate that this type of technology is likely to be both complex and costly (as opposed to *high technology*, which makes it possible to treat disease successfully, based on a genuine understanding of the disease mechanism and which is usually less costly and easier to deliver). A discussion of the role of the PA catheter in the performance of this complicated procedure seems particularly apt since both of these procedures have had a profound impact on the therapy of disease [5], have been widely and perhaps overly accepted at a significant financial and social cost, and, upon reaching a certain point, have been subjected to serious scrutiny. Thus, the risk–benefit ratios and cost effectiveness of both of these procedures have been questioned.

Each of the three major randomized clinical studies comparing CABG sur-gery to medical therapy (CASS, ECSS, and the VA) has generated heated debate, and each has been criticized extensively. However, despite the methodologic differences between them, Killip and Ryan [6] believe that certain conclusions regarding patient selection for CABG are warranted. Their conclusions are that bypass surgery appears to offer a significant sur-vival advantage in patients with hemodynamically significant left main dis-ease, in patients with three-vessel disease and impaired ventricular function (ejection fraction generally below 0.50), and possibly in patients in certain other high-risk subgroups (defined in the VA and ECSS studies) which include peripheral vascular disease, marked ST segment depression on exercise testing, abnormal resting electrocardiogram (ECG), increasing age, previous myocar-dial infarction, and hypertension. Concerning patients to be excluded from surgery, they note that surgery can be safely postponed in the patient who is functioning well despite ischemic symptoms until he no longer responds to maximal medical therapy. Specifically, that surgery does not alter long-term survival and the occurrence of reinfarction in low-risk patients will ensure that patients presenting for surgery will only be medical therapy failures on maximal doses of medication and not low-risk patients hoping for either a survival advantage or for prophylaxis against future myocardial infarction. These conclusions are likely to be increasingly accepted by the majority of referring cardiologists in this country, especially since the clinician now has newer modes of medical therapy (calcium channel blockers) as well as an attractive option that was not available previously, namely, PTCA. This procedure, which is closer to the definition of *high technology* is significantly less expensive than CABG ($5000–$7000 per patient) [2] and is being widely adopted in this country [7]. As cardiologists become more proficient and comfortable performing PTCA, it is being applied to patients at higher risk, including those with totally occluded vessels [8] as well as those with partially occluded saphenous vein grafts [9]. Given strong economic pressure from both government and insurance carriers to reduce health care costs, as well as the widespread acceptance of PTCA by "interventional" cardiologists competing with surgeons for their share of the dwindling health-care dollar, we believe that the number of low-risk patients presenting for CABG surgery will continue to decline. Results from the major studies, however, suggest that CABG surgery may prolong survival in elderly (those over 65 years) high-risk patients [10].

Based on these studies, it is clear that anesthesiologists will be increasingly called upon to care for high-risk patients with moderate-to-severe reductions of ventricular function, with prior myocardial infarction and associated degrees of ventricular dyssynergy, and who are refractory to medical therapy, PTCA, or both. An increasing number of patients will be elderly, have other significant intercurrent medical illnesses, and may present for "redo" CABG or simultaneous valve replacement, which carries higher operative mortality [11]. This patient profile, that of a progressively increasing number of preoperative risk factors, has been the experience at our institution (San Francisco Veterans Administration Medical Center, University of California, San Francisco) and has been substantiated, as recently reported by Cosgrove et al., in a large-scale analysis of 24,672 patients operated on at the Cleveland Clinic from 1970 to 1982 [12].

ARGUMENT 2

PA monitoring has been shown to provide valuable hemodynamic data not obtainable by physical examination or CVP monitoring. When properly measured and analyzed, these data have been shown to be a valuable adjunct to clinical care. The use of the PA catheter during CABG surgery provides assistance in the safe induction and maintenance of anesthesia, the detection of perioperative myocardial ischemia, and determination of the "optimal" cardiac output and mean arterial pressure (MAP) compatible with safe termination of cardiopulmonary bypass (CPB). It is also a necessary guide to the rational perioperative use of inotropes, vasopressors, and vasodilators.

The poor correlation of CVP with left-sided filling pressures (pulmonary artery wedge pressure [PAWP] and left ventricular end-diastolic pressure [LVEDP]) has been well documented along with the potential danger in using CVP measurements alone to guide the diagnosis and therapy of critically ill medical and surgical patients [13–16]. Although most clinicians would not dispute these facts, which specific groups of patients either require (for diagnosis of illness) or will benefit from (for guidance of therapy and improvement of outcome) PA monitoring remains to be resolved. Over the past several years, large-scale prospective randomized clinical trials have been performed comparing CVP to PA monitoring to determine the risk–benefit ratios [17] and, most importantly, their value in altering patient outcome [18, 19]. While we do not dispute the need for such trials and welcome investigators willing to undergo the arduous task of dealing with the multiplicity of variables that have to be controlled when studying a large number of critically ill patients, several recent studies have inferred (but not definitively proved) that PA monitoring in the intensive-care setting is a valuable adjunct to diagnosis and guidance of therapy. Connors et al. [20] prospectively studied 62 right-heart catheterizations in critically ill medical patients without evidence of recent myocardial infarction, and found that physicians' estimates of hemodynamic variables based on the physical examination were frequently in error and, more importantly, that the results of the catheterization frequently resulted in changes in therapy. Accurate prediction of hemodynamics was poor, ranging from 42% correct for PAWP to 44% correct for cardiac index (CI) and mean PA pressure. There were no significant differences in the accuracy of predictions made by attendings, fellows, or residents. Based on the results of catheterization, changes in therapy were made in 48% of cases, although the general outcome was poor with a 57% mortality rate. Similar results were obtained by Eisenberg et al. [21] (a 30% correct prediction of PAWP, 50% for CI, systemic vascular resistance [SVR], or right atrial pressure, with alteration of therapy in 58%). Shoemaker has shown that the use of PA catheterization as part of an aggressive therapeutic protocol to limit the overall oxygen debt through optimization of systemic oxygen transport and cardiac output significantly reduces the overall complication and mortality rate in a prospective randomized group of medical/surgical intensive-care-unit patients (W.C. Shoemaker, personal communication, 1986). Simply achieving normality of either PAWP or CVP did not alter outcome.

The value of PA monitoring during CABG surgery has been appreciated by the cardiac surgeon. Although no studies specifically address the issue in isolation, a number of cardiac surgeons believe that improvements in intraoperative anesthetic techniques along with the routine use of cold cardioplegia for myocardial preservation have been responsible for the substantial decrease in morbidity and mortality associated with CABG surgery that has been noted since the early 1970s [12, 22–25]. The addition of advanced hemodynamic monitoring to the armamentarium of the cardiac anesthetist must be included as a major factor in improving intraoperative anesthetic technique.

The first major study in the anesthesia literature addressing the potential utility (or lack thereof) of PA monitoring in patients undergoing CABG surgery was performed by Mangano [16]. This study addressed a specific physiologic question: what is the correlation of CVP and PAWP before, during, and after CABG surgery? This study included patients with impaired preoperative ventricular function and angiographic evidence of dyssynergy, excluding patients with valvular heart disease or ventricular aneurysms. Although not specifically excluded, no patient had cor pulmonale, elevations of pulmonary vascular resistance, or pulmonary hypertension. The results demonstrated that two distinct patient groups exhibited significant differences in their patterns of CVP and PAWP correlation. In patients with ejection fractions greater than 0.50 and without angiographic evidence of dyssynergy, the absolute values of CVP and PAWP correlated well ($r = 0.89$) during the 36 h study period, as did relative changes in both variables ($r = 0.94$). However, in patients with ejection fractions less than 0.40 or with dyssynergy, the correlation was poor ($r = 0.24$) and the change in CVP did not correlate with the change in pulmonary capillary wedge pressure (PCWP) ($r = 0.04$). Normality of the CVP was predictive of normality of the PAWP in only 65% of data points. The correlation improved significantly following bypass in 40% of the patients, which may reflect the early (often immediate) improvement of regional wall motion and systolic thickening noted on transesophageal echo-cardiography by Topol et al. following successful revascularization [26]. However, the fact that 60% of these patients failed to improve (30% of the total study group) indicates clearly that the majority of high-risk patients are at substantial jeopardy for "uninformed" therapeutic decision making by the clinician. Although this study only examined the use of the PA catheter for estimation of preload, we believe that the importance of utilizing several parameters influencing cardiac function including estimates of loading conditions (PAWP, MAP, and SVR), contractility and pump function (cardiac output, stroke volume, stroke work), and systemic oxygen delivery cannot be over-emphasized when managing the patient undergoing CABG surgery.

In contrast to the number of studies in the intensive-care literature documenting the utility of PA monitoring in guiding clinical care, there is a paucity of studies in the anesthesia literature specifically addressing this question. Although the physiologic study by Mangano was interpreted by many to indicate that PA monitoring was of limited value in the majority of patients presenting for CABG surgery [27], in point of fact, here at our institution, PA lines are used routinely because we rarely see a patient who meets the definition of what others may call "low risk".

Waller et al. [28, 29] reported preliminary data on the utility of PA monitoring in patients with normal left ventricular function undergoing "routine"

CABG. Of the 15 patients studied, the correlation of CVP with PAWP was poor ($r < 0.6$) in nine patients and good in only one ($r = 0.86$). Staff anesthesiologists, blinded to all data routinely obtained by PA monitoring with the exception of CVP, were noted to be unaware of what were termed *severe* hemodynamic abnormalities (PCWP > 15–20, PCWP "V" waves > 20–25, CI < 1.5, and SVR > 2500) 65% of the time that these abnormalities were present. Furthermore, abnormalities of these variables occurred in 87% of patients (34% before intubation and 54% before skin incision). The clinicians were notified immediately of severe abnormalities in order to institute therapy. It is presumed that these patients did well, which has been used as an argument to weaken the importance of the study, yet the fact that the severe abnormalities were unblinded by the investigator could have biased the outcomes. Thus, it would appear that abnormalities of hemodynamics that may be potentially life threatening and are clinically silent (presumably until the point of bad outcome) are common and can be detected by PA monitoring. However, it appears that we must await further clinical studies to validate and extend this contention. In addition, this study has been used by some to justify preinduction placement of PA catheters (which we support). This issue has been well summarized elsewhere [30, 31].

A recent report presented retrospectively obtained outcome data from low-risk patients (ejection fraction > 40–50%, no history of congestive heart failure, and normal arterial blood pressure response to exercise testing) undergoing CABG to support the contention that CVP monitoring alone is adequate. Bashein et al. [32] analyzed consecutive cases monitored with CVP alone from 1981 to 1983 and noted that, of 698 "low-risk" cases, there was an in-hospital mortality of 0.72% and a perioperative infarction rate of <2.06%. However, postoperative PA monitoring was subsequently thought to be necessary in 4.7%, and two patients had severe intraoperative complications, requiring more sophisticated monitoring than CVP. Given that the PA catheter utilization rate in the total population at that time was 45.3%, with the addition of the low-risk patients requiring PA monitoring, the average utilization rate rose to 50%. We would expect that more recent analysis would yield an even higher utilization rate, given the increasing risk profile of CABG patients over time. Thus, it would appear that the PA catheter seems to be a rather well-established "routine" monitoring tool at Bashein's institution.

In addition to the data presented above, there would appear to be other potential theoretical benefits for the use of the PA catheter to guide the induction and maintenance of anesthesia in CABG patients. Wynands et al. [33], studying patients anesthetized with fentanyl–oxygen that had impaired left ventricular function, demonstrated that significant increases in SVR (17%–81%), associated with decreases in CI (12%–36%), occurred in the absence of changes in MAP and PAWP during sternotomy and aortic dissection in six of the seven patients. Nitrous oxide has been shown to act similarly in patients with preoperative elevations of LVEDP (>15 mmHg) when added to a fentanyl–oxygen anesthetic [34]. These studies stress the potential benefit of monitoring additional physiologic parameters in guiding anesthetic management.

Recent studies by Rao et al. [35] and Slogoff and Keats [36] suggest that PA monitoring can play a significant role in lowering the perioperative infarction rate. The study by Rao et al. demonstrated the utility of rigorous detection and therapy of abnormal hemodynamic values in reducing the reinfarction rate in patients undergoing noncardiac surgery. Using this approach, they reduced the perioperative reinfarction rate from 7.7% in a retrospective control group to 1.9% in their prospective cohort. Of the 733 prospective patients, 83% were monitored with PA catheters. Patients who had elevations of PAWP greater than 25 mmHg at anytime during the perioperative period had a 28% incidence of reinfarction. Slogoff and Keats found that ECG evidence of perioperative myocardial ischemia during elective CABG was significantly associated with a threefold increase in the postoperative infarction rate (6.9% vs 2.5%). Although this study did not investigate the effects of therapy of this ischemia on outcome, and the use of PA monitoring in this group was not discussed, it does point out the potential impact of detecting myocardial ischemia. Both of these studies have generated considerable controversy and await further validation, but the basic tenets are generally well accepted by most clinicians.

The increase in left ventricular filling pressure that commonly accompanies ischemia results from a combination of factors, including a reduction of diastolic distensibility as well as a component of systolic dysfunction [37]. Sasayama et al. [38], studying pacing-induced ischemia, demonstrated that this increase is primarily a result of an upward shift of the ischemic myocardial segments pressure–segment length relation. Furthermore, the increase in diastolic stretch of the nonischemic myocardium is an important compensatory mechanism that allows preservation of stroke volume despite decreased systolic shortening of the ischemic segment. Thus, it is believed that the ultimate increase in ventricular end–diastolic pressure is a result of this "variable diastolic compliance". It is clear that this response is a complex interplay of different factors and may very according to the type of ischemia present (decreases in supply or increases in demand).

The value of the PA catheter as a monitor of myocardial ischemia has been popularized by Kaplan and Wells [39], who presented data supporting the concept that intraoperative ischemic responses are similar to those noted in the cardiac cath lab. They found that abnormalities of the PAWP tracing suggestive of ischemia (abnormal AC wave > 15 torr, V wave > 20 torr) occurred in 55% of the patients thought to have developed ischemia. ST segment changes were present in only 44%. As noted in the cath lab, elevations of PAWP commonly preceded changes in the ST segment by several minutes [40]. They were unable to correlate these changes in compliance with either the number of vessels diseased or the degree of ventricular dysfunction. A recent study by Tarnow et al. [41], examining the effects of isoflurane–nitrous oxide anesthesia on the threshold to pacing-induced ischemia in CABG patients, documented the appearance of prominent PCWP "V" waves in 89% of patients who developed ECG signs of ischemia. Abnormal CVP "V" waves occurred in only 22% of patients.

Although abnormalities of regional segmental wall motion, detected by transesophageal echocardiography, have been shown to be more sensitive than the intraoperative ECG [42], the prohibitive cost and lack of on-line analysis of present echo systems make it a less accessible and useful tool to the vast majority of clinicians. In addition, interpreting the ECG in patients with conduction abnormalities, taking digoxin, in the face of axis shifts, etc., is often difficult or impossible. The monitoring of PAWP, although it may reflect a complex interplay of factors, provides important diagnostic and often confirmatory information regarding the presence of myocardial ischemia that is only rarely obtainable with CVP monitoring. This information, when properly interpreted and acted upon, may lead to more favorable patient outcomes.

Discontinuation and weaning from cardiopulmonary bypass is a hazardous time for the patient and, for the clinician, it is by far the most challenging time period during CABG surgery. It requires close attention to and utilization of as much hemodynamic information as the clinician is capable of using for intelligent diagnostic and therapeutic decision making. The patient may or may not have undergone successful revascularization, depending on the coronary anatomy as well as the technical skill of the surgeon. Cardiac protection may have been inadequate due to the presence of severe stenosis, limiting the distribution of cardioplegia. Impairment of coronary autoregulation and myocardial edema can potentially result in impairment of cellular integrity and function.

Mangano [43] and others [44–46] have documented that ventricular function is depressed often to profound levels both early and late in the perioperative period following myocardial revascularization. In a group of 22 patients studied by Mangano, eight sets of left and right ventricular function curves (LVFC and RVFC) were generated by altering preload (by changing body position) during the 24 h perioperative period following pericardiotomy. Depression of ventricular function, ranging from 35% to 75% of control, occurred in all patients at 15 min following bypass. In patients with preoperative ejection fractions of less than 0.45 or with angiographic evidence of dyssynergy, the depression was most profound (depression of LVFC and RVFC to 40% and 30% of control, respectively) and persisted for 24 h after revascularization. Patients in this group recovered to only 60% of control at 24 h. Patients with normal preoperative ventricular function exhibited recovery to 90% of control within 4 h after termination of bypass. Statistically significant differences in PAWP pressure were noted between the two groups at 15 min, 1 h, and 2 h after bypass (with the higher PAWPs in the impaired ventricular function group). Poor correlation of CVP and PAWP is suggested by the fact that there were no significant differences noted in CVP between groups during these time periods. The ventricular function curves exhibited relatively flat slopes. This has been reported previously in studies performed at this institution in which PAWP, end-diastolic volume, and ejection fraction using first-pass radio-nuclide techniques were measured during volume loading following bypass [47, 48]. Little augmentation of stroke volume occurred above a PCWP of 7 mmHg or an end-diastolic volume index of 70 ml/m². In addition, although increases in preload resulted in increases in ventricular output, ejection fraction fell progressively. This fall in ejection fraction may result in over-distention of the left ventricle, which could be accompanied by deleterious increases in myocardial oxygen consumption. Thus, although the PAWP may be an unreliable indicator of ventricular volume, avoiding excessive elevation of PAWP at termination of bypass may result in the most favorable conditions for overall ventricular oxygen demand during this critical time. This cannot be accomplished using CVP alone, as significant elevations of PAWP may be present with a low or normal CVP.

Without the aid of the PA catheter, the clinician has only a limited amount of information with which to evaluate cardiac and circulatory function: the CVP and the surgeon's palpation of the pulmonary artery may be used to evaluate preload, the configuration of the arterial waveform may be used as an estimate of contractility and SVR, the value of the MAP may be used as an overall measure of function, and the base deficit on the arterial blood gas may be used as an overall measure of oxygen delivery and utilization by the tissues. These can provide a substantial amount of information in the patient with good preoperative ventricular function and favorable coronary anatomy, and who is operated on by a skillful surgeon during a short period of aortic cross-clamping. It may be all that is needed for decision making in the majority of these patients. However, this is inadequate for the high-risk patients that we encounter. The surgeon's finger on the PA is very likely the same one that was unable to perform the best possible revascularization, thus leaving the patient in substantial jeopardy. Estimation of preload may be grossly inaccurate. Overzealous volume loading may lead to decreases in ejection fraction and overdistention of the ventricle with attendant obligatory increases in oxygen demand. The arterial waveform may also be an inaccurate guide of therapy as has been demonstrated in a recent study by Gerber et al. [49], who were unable to find any significant correlation between SVR and the height of the dicrotic notch, the slope of the diastolic runoff, or stroke volume. Neither could cardiac output or stroke volume be correlated with the height of the dicrotic notch. The direct measurement of SVR using thermodilution cardiac outputs is the only widely accepted method to obtain SVR currently available.

These studies highlight the value of PA monitoring in optimizing cardiac output and MAP, utilizing the lowest possible PAWP at which "normal values" occur in order to avoid overdistention of a depressed and vulnerable myocardium following bypass. Utilization of CVP only to guide volume infusion therapy is inadequate given the additional fact that the right ventricular function is significantly depressed [43, 50], with a separate and independent set of moderating factors (i.e., changes in pulmonary vascular resistance due to loss of lung volume, effects of hypothermia on pulmonary compliance, inadequate protection due to rapid rewarming, etc.). The variable changes that may be encountered in SVR, which are very difficult to detect by physical examination even when the clinician has access to more than the patient's head, make the use of MAP alone as an endpoint for "homeostasis" similarly inadequate. We believe that measuring and attempting to optimize several important physiologic factors (such as cardiac output, SVR and pulmonary vascular resistance [PVR], and MAP) which, although interrelated physiologically, may be therapeutically independent, is the most rational way to manage patients in the early (and late) time period following cardiopulmonary bypass.

ARGUMENT 3

The additional cost of PA over CVP monitoring is insignificant when compared to the overall cost of CABG surgery. In fact, it may result in lower cost if it assists in the diagnosis or therapy of postoperative complications, allowing shorter intensive-care stay. CABG surgery is expensive, ranging from $15,000 to $25,000 per patient. Whether or not PA monitoring adds substantial expense or may actually save money by allowing more effective therapy and diagnosis of complications of surgery or anesthesia is an important issue. To support our contention that the additional cost of PA monitoring over the placement of a CVP catheter is negligible when compared to the overall cost of the surgery and to dispel the notion that eliminating routine PA monitoring would result in significant cost savings, it is necessary to examine what data there are on cost containment in CABG surgery. Estimating the actual added cost of PA over CVP monitoring, including the cost of the catheter, insertion time, cost of other hardware necessary to maintain the catheter and derive hemodynamic information from it, is difficult and varies according to the type of hospital and its billing practices. The cost of a PA catheter (with capability for thermodilution output) ranges from $100 to $150 while the cost of a CVP catheter is probably one-third to one-fifth of that. At the University of California, San Francisco, our Anesthesia Department includes the insertion of a PA catheter in the startup charge for complicated surgical procedures such as CABG or major vascular surgery. For cases in which it would not be expected to be a routine part of anesthetic management, a separate modest charge is assessed. In the intensive-care unit, there is no additional charge for obtaining the additional hemodynamic data available from the PA catheter (although there is a charge for the small amount of additional hardware necessary) (N.H. Cohen, personal communication, 1986). We can conservatively estimate that, all factors included, the cost of PA monitoring over CVP ranges from $250 to $750. Given the overall cost of CABG surgery (using the range of $20,000–

$25,000), these charges would account for no less than 1% to no more than 3.75% of the total.

The few studies that have specifically addressed cost containment in cardiac surgery have looked at small numbers of patients, analyzed practices at a limited number of hospitals (usually only the authors' primary affiliation), and excluded "sick" patients from consideration. Tomatis et al. [51] analyzed the cost of 30 cardiac operations (ten of which were CABG surgery) at a community hospital. By discussing the charges with the responsible department and personnel, the authors attempted to reduce them by "expense rationalization". By reducing room charges through later admission and earlier discharge from the intensive-care unit, the elimination of postoperative IPPB therapy, fewer routine lab tests, and elimination of "routine" use of high-dose steroids after induction of anesthesia "to prevent pump lung" (this alone accounted for almost 20% of the total savings), they were able to reduce overall charges by only 11%. Operating-room charges accounted for about 40% of the bill, while surgeons' fees accounted for 27%. Loop et al. [52] analyzed the cost of hospitalization of 25 patients admitted the morning of surgery (as opposed to the usual 2 days prior to surgery). By reducing length of stay, decreasing the period of intensive care, practicing blood conservation (including elimination of routine cross-matching), and eliminating the routine use of the PA catheter in patients with normal ventricular function, they were only able to realize a 10% reduction in overall charge. Egdahl [53], in an accompanying editorial, makes two significant points. First, that due to "elasticity of demand", decreasing unit costs may actually result in increased utilization of services and thus overall increases in cost. More importantly, he notes that surgeons' (and to a lesser degree other professional) fees are the major source of expense, accounting for 30%–40% of the total bill. He notes that cardiac surgical fees are among the highest in medicine and that they were set as such when cardiac procedures carried higher mortality, required longer operating time, and the patient required more primary care by the surgeon alone. He makes the presumably unpopular suggestion that they should be reduced, reflecting the fact that mortality is now lower, operations shorter, and more material and personnel support are available to the surgeon (although there is no mention of the impact of the malpractice crisis!). In a more recent cost study by Vander Salm and Blair [54], the topic of surgeons' fees was not addressed.

With regard to the increasing provision of CABG surgery to older groups of patients, Roberts et al. [4] retrospectively analyzed morbidity and mortality, length of hospital stay, and cost in old (>65 years) and young (<60 years). They found that, although early (30 day) mortality was similar between groups, 120 day mortality was higher in the elderly (7.6% vs 1.3%). The elderly patients suffered more complications and had longer intensive-care and total hospital stay. The average cost for the younger group was $18,000 as opposed to $28,000 for the elderly. All patients received "close hemodynamic monitoring" for at least 48 h postoperatively. Although the value of such monitoring is only implied, if it leads to fewer complications or more efficient therapy of new complications or preexisting medical illness, actual cost savings could be realized.

The overall conclusions reached by these studies are similar to those reported by Showstack et al. of a larger-scale study assessing the role of changing clinical practices on the overall cost of health care [3]. Looking at 2011 patients hospitalized at the University of California, San Francisco, over the period from 1972 to 1982, they demonstrated that neither "little ticket" technology (small procedures, widely and easily utilized, and less expensive technologies such as laboratory tests) nor "big ticket" technology (large-scale expensive technology such as computed tomographic scanners and renal dialysis) [55] contributed significantly to the overall rise in health costs. The major offender was the increasing provision of surgery to larger groups of critically ill patients (such as CABG surgery to patients with acute myocardial infarction, ligation of patent ductus arteriosus to premature babies, and cesarean sections). Thus, it would appear that, when fixed hospital charges and professional fees are assessed, the role of the PA catheter in the overall cost of health care is minimal. Furthermore, that it is the increasing provision of the operation itself that accounts for such great expense would indicate that the most effective way to decrease costs is either to decrease the number of operations being performed or, if the operation is going to be performed, to take all steps necessary to ensure that it is done as safely as possible to avoid complications. We believe that the provision of PA monitoring, when done properly, is a way to increase patient safety and treat the patient based on the maximum amount of knowledge that is currently routinely available.

ARGUMENT 4

PA monitoring, performed by personnel with skill and experience, especially when used for short periods of time, is a safe procedure with a very low complication rate. A number of serious, life-threatening complications are as likely to occur with the use of CVP monitoring.

The complications of PA monitoring have been reviewed in a number of publications encompassing a variety of critically ill patients [14, 56, 57]. It is clear that a number of complications, ranging in incidence and severity from transient premature ventricular contractions on insertion (which are very common and usually insignificant) to pulmonary artery rupture (which is very rare and life threatening), can occur. Some complications, such as those related to venous cannulation (carotid artery puncture, pneumothorax) are as common an occurrence with CVP as with PA monitoring. Embolic and thrombotic complications may occur, but have probably been reduced with the use of heparin-bonded catheters [58]. Right-sided endocardial damage, including sterile or septic hemmorrhage or thrombus, occurs primarily in debilitated patients who are bacteremic and monitored for prolonged periods of time [59]. Life-threatening symptomatic arrhythmias, such as sustained ventricular tachycardia or fibrillation, also occur primarily in critically ill patients in the intensive care unit. It has been noted that some of the necessary accompaniments of cardiopulmonary bypass, namely, anticoagulation, hypothermia, nonventilated deflated lungs, and a surgeon manipulating the heart, pose a particular hazard for pulmonary artery rupture. During hypothermic bypass, distal migration of a stiffer catheter [60] through empty cardiac chambers into a more brittle pulmonary vasculature can result in rupture by "puncture" or by cracking of the vessel wall with balloon inflation. Hemorrhage of cold heparinized blood may be very difficult to control. However, this complication is rare and it is likely to become even less common as the postulated mechanisms are investigated (including that of the pressure generated by balloon inflation in a variety of models) [61], and simple recommendations for prophylaxis (withdrawing the catheter 5 cm just before bypass or not inflating the balloon while on bypass or before a typical PA trace is present) as well as for therapy (application of 20 cm H_2O PEEP to the airway or immediate pulmonary resection if bleeding is severe) are followed. Two large-scale prospective studies of complication rates have documented the low incidence of morbidity or mortality associated with PA monitoring in surgical populations. Shah et al. [62] reported on 6245 catheterizations performed from 1977 to 1982. Only one death occurred in a patient in which 5 ml of air was used to inflate the balloon, resulting in PA rupture. Three PA ruptures occurred on bypass, all of which were controlled with PEEP only. Boyd et al. [63] reported on 500 consecutive patients catheterized in 1981. "Serious" complications (ventricular tachycardia, septicemia, pulmonary infiltrates, or pulmonary hemorrhage) occurred in 4.4% of catheterizations, yet only one patient developed PA rupture (which was nonfatal). Given this low rate of complications, it is significant that 80% of the physicians caring for these patients found the information obtained from the catheter either "very helpful" or "helpful." Thus, it appears that most, if not all, or the major clinically significant complications of both PA and CVP monitoring are preventable with proper training in techniques of insertion, appreciation of all the components of the monitoring system, and knowledge of how they are affected by the "environment" of the operating room and intensive care unit. In addition, it is the responsibility of the clinician to ensure that less skilled personnel who may be using the catheter as part of the patient's care are properly educated. There is no substitute for, nor escaping of the anesthesiologists' credo: "Vigilance".

REFERENCES

1. Pluth JR: Operative mortality and morbidity for initial and repeat coronary artery bypass grafting [editorial]. Ann Thorac Surg 38:552–553, 1984.
2. Lenfant C, Roth CA: Advances in cardiology and escalating costs to the patient: a view from the government [editorial]. Circulation 71:424–428, 1985.

3. Showstack JA, Stone MH, Schroeder SA: The role of changing clinical practices in the rising costs of hospital care. N Engl J Med 313:1201–1207, 1985.
4. Roberts AJ, Woodhall DD, Conti CR, Ellison DW, Fisher R, Richards C, Marks RG, Knauf DG, Alexander JA: Mortality, morbidity, and cost-accounting related to coronary artery bypass graft surgery in the elderly. Ann Thorac Surg 39:426–432, 1985.
5. Swan HJC, Ganz W: Hemodynamic mesurements in clinical practice: a decade in review. J Am Coll Cardiol 1:103–113, 1983.
6. Killip T, Ryan TJ: Randomized trials in coronary bypass surgery [editorial]. Circulation 71:418–421, 1985.
7. Kent KM, Bentivoglio LG, Block PC, Bourassa MG, Cowley MJ, Dorros G, Detre KM, Gosselin AJ, Gruentzig AR, Kelsey SF: Long-term efficacy of percutaneous transluminal coronary angioplasty (PTCA): report from the National Heart, Lung, and Blood Institute PTCA Registry. Am J Cardiol 53:27C–31C, 1984.
8. Kereiakes DJ, Selmon MR, McAuley BJ, McAuley DB, Sheehan DJ, Simpson JB: Angioplasty in total coronary artery occlusion: experience in 76 consecutive patients. J Am Coll Cardiol 6:526–533, 1985.
9. Dorros G, Johnson WD, Tector AJ, Schmahl TM, Kalush SL, Janke L: Percutaneous transluminal coronary angioplasty in patients with prior coronary artery bypass grafting. J Thorac Cardiovasc Surg 87:17–26, 1984.
10. Gersh BJ, Kronmal RA, Schaff HV, Frye RL, Ryan TJ, Mock MB, Myers WO, Athearn MW, Gosselin AJ, Kaiser GC, Bourassa MG, Killip III T, et al.: Comparison of coronary artery bypass surgery and medical therapy in patients 65 years of age or older. N Engl J Med 313:217–224, 1985.
11. Schaff HV, Orszulak TA, Gersh BJ, Piehler JM, Puga FJ, Danielson GK, Pluth JR: The morbidity and mortality of reoperation for coronary artery disease and analysis of late results with use of actuarial estimate of event-free interval. J Thorac Cardiovasc Surg 85:508–515, 1983.
12. Cosgrove DM, Loop FD, Lytle BW, Baillot R, Gill CC, Golding LAR, Taylor PC, Goormastic M: Primary myocardial revascularization: trends in surgical mortality. J Thorac Cardiovasc Surg 88:673–684, 1984.
13. Swan HJC, Ganz W: Measurement of right atrial and pulmonary arterial pressures and cardiac output: clinical application of hemodynamic monitoring. Adv Intern Med 27:453–473, 1982.
14. Pace NL: A critique of flow-directed pulmonary arterial catheterization. Anesthesiology 47:455–465, 1977.
15. Manny J, Grindlinger GA, Dennis RC, Weisel RD, Hechtman HB: Myocardial performance curves as guide to volume therapy. Surg Gynecol Obstet 149:863–873, 1979.
16. Mangano DT: Monitoring pulmonary arterial pressure in coronary-artery disease. Anesthesiology 53:364–370, 1980.
17. Spodick DH: Physiologic and prognostic implications of invasive monitoring: undetermined risk/benefit ratios in patients with heart disease [editorial]. Am J Cardiol 46:173–175, 1980.
18. Robin ED: Cult of the Swan–Ganz catheter: overuse and abuse of pulmonary flow catheters. Ann Intern Md 103:445–449, 1985.
19. Keefer JR, Barash PG: Pulmonary artery catheterization: a decade of clinical progress? [editorial] Chest 84:241–242, 1983.
20. Connors AF, McCaffree DR, Gray BA: Evaluation of right-heart catheterization in the critically ill patient without acute myocardial infarction. N Engl J Med 308:263–267, 1983.
21. Eisenberg PR, Jaffe AS, Schuster DP: Clinical evaluation compared to pulmonary artery catheterization in the hemodynamic assessment of critically ill patients. Crit Care Med 12:549–553, 1984.
22. Kouchoukos NT, Oberman A, Kirklin JW, Russell RO Jr, Karp RB, Pacifico AD, Zorn GL: Coronary bypass surgery: analysis of factors affecting hospital mortality. Circulation [Suppl 1] 62:184–189, 1980.
23. Theman TE, Reid D: Circulatory support after coronary artery surgery. Can J Surg 26:233–235, 1983.
24. Moore CH, Lombardo TR, Allums JA, Gordon FT: Left main coronary artery stenosis: hemodynamic monitoring to reduce mortality. Ann Thorac Surg 26:445–451, 1978.
25. Roberts AJ: Perioperative myocardial infarction and changes in left ventricular performance related to coronary artery bypass graft surgery. Ann Thorac Surg 35:208–225, 1983.
26. Topol EJ, Weiss JL, Guzman PA, Dorsey-Lima S, Blanck TJJ, Humphrey LS, Baumgartner

WA, Flaherty JT, Reitz BA: Immediate improvement of dysfunctional myocardial segments after coronary revascularization: detection by intraoperative transesophageal echocardiography. J Am Coll Cardiol 4:1123–1134, 1984.

27. Lowenstein E, Teplick R: To (PA) catheterize or not to (PA) catheterize: that is the question [editorial]. Anesthesiology 53:361–363, 1980.

28. Waller JL, Johnson SP, Kaplan JA: Usefulness of pulmonary artery catheters during aortocoronary bypass surgery [abstr]. Anesth Analg 61:221–222, 1982.

29. Waller JL, Johnson SP, kalpan JA, Craver JM: Usefulness of puomonary [sic] artery catheters during aortocoronary bypass surgery [abstr]. Am J Cardiol 49:907, 1982.

30. Streisand JB, Clark NJ, Pace NL: Placement of the pulmonary arterial catheter before anesthesia for cardiac surgery: safe, intelligent, and appropriate use of invasive hemodynamic monitoring. J Clin Monit 1:193–196, 1985.

31. Dzelzkalns R, Stanley TH: Placement of the pulmonary arterial catheter before anesthesia for cardiac surgery: a stressful, painful, unnecessary crutch. J Clin Monit 1:197–200, 1985.

32. Bashein G, Johnson PW, Davis KB, Ivey TD: Elective coronary bypass surgery without pulmonary artery catheter monitoring. Anesthesiology 63:451–454, 1985.

33. Wynands JE, Wong P, Whalley DG, Sprigge JS, Townsend GE, Patel YC: Oxygen–fentanyl anesthesia in patients with poor left ventricular function: hemodynamics and plasma fentanyl concentrations. Anesth Analg 62:476–482, 1983.

34. Balasaraswathi K, Kumar P, Rao TLK, El-Etr AA: Left ventricular end-diastolic pressure (LVEDP) as an index for nitrous oxide use during coronary artery surgery. Anesthesiology 55:708–709, 1981.

35. Rao TLK, Jacobs KH, El-Etr AA: Reinfarction following anesthesia in patients with myocardial infarction. Anesthesiology 59:499–505, 1983.

36. Slogoff S, Keats AS: Does perioperative myocardial ischemia lead to postoperative myocardial infarction? Anesthesiology 62:107–114, 1985.

37. Grossman W: Why is left ventricular diastolic pressure increased during angina pectoris [editorial]. J Am Coll Cardiol 5:607–608, 1985.

38. Sasayama S, Nonogi H, Miyazaki S, Sakurai T, Kawai C, Eiho S, Kuwahara M: Changes in diastolic properties of the regional myocardium during pacing-induced ischemia in human subjects. J Am Coll Cardiol 5:599–606, 1985.

39. Kaplan JA, Wells PH: Early diagnosis of myocardial ischemia using the pulmonary arterial catheter. Anesth Analg 60:789–793, 1981.

40. Doorey AJ, Mehmel HC, Schwarz FX, Kubler W: Amelioration by nitroglycerin of left ventricular ischemia induced by percutaneous transluminal coronary angioplasty: assessment by hemodynamic variables and left ventriculography. J Am Coll Cardiol 6:267–274, 1985.

41. Tarnow J, Markschies-Hornung A, Schulte-Sasse U: Isoflurane improves the tolerance to pacing-induced myocardial ischemia. Anesthesiology 64:147–156, 1986.

42. Smith JS, Cahalan MK, Benefiel DJ, Byrd BF, Lurz FW, Shapiro WA, Roizen MF, Bouchard A, Schiller NB: Intraoperative detection of myocardial ischemia in high-risk patients: electrocardiography versus two-dimensional transesophageal echocardiography. Circulation 72: 1015–1021, 1985.

43. Mangano DT: Biventricular function after myocardial revascularization in humans: deterioration and recovery patterns during the first 24 hours. Anesthesiology 62:571–577, 1985.

44. Gray R, Maddahi J, Berman D, Raymond M, Waxman A, Ganz W, Matloff J, Swan HJC: Scintigraphic and hemodynamic demonstration of transient left ventricular dysfunction immediately after uncomplicated coronary artery bypass grafting. J Thorac Cardiovasc Surg 77:504–510, 1979.

45. Roberts AJ, Spies SM, Meyers SN, Moran JM, Sanders JH Jr, Lichtenthal PR, Michaelis LL: Early and long-term improvement in left ventricular performance following coronary bypass surgery. Surgery 88:467–475, 1980.

46. Fremes SE, Weisel RD, Mickle DAG, Ivanov J, Madonik MM, Seawright SJ, Houle S, McLaughlin PR, Baird RJ: Myocardial metabolism and ventricular function following cold potassium cardioplegia. J Thorac Cardiovasc Surg 89:531–546, 1985.

47. Mangano DT, Van Dyke DC, Ellis RJ: The effect of increasing preload on ventricular output and ejection in man: limitations of the Frank–Starling mechanism. Circulation 62:535–541, 1980.

48. Ellis RJ, Mangano DT, Van Dyke DC: Relationship of wedge pressure to end-diastolic

volume in patients undergoing myocardial revascularization. J Thorac Cardiovasc Surg 78:605–613, 1979.

49. Gerber MJ, Carp D, Hines R, Barash PG: Arterial waveforms and systemic vascular resistance: is there a correlation? [abstr] Anesthesiology 63:A70, 1985.
50. Christakis GT, Fremes SE, Weisel RD, Ivanov J, Madonik MM, Seawright SJ, McLaughlin PR: Right ventricular dysfunction following cold potassium carioplegia. J Thorac Cardiovasc Surg 90:243–250, 1985.
51. Tomatis LA, Schlosser RJ, Riahi M, Stockinger FL, Kanten R: Cost containment via expense rationalization in open-heart surgery. J Thorac Cardiovasc Surg 77:448–451, 1979.
52. Loop FD, Christiansen EK, Lester JL, Cosgrove DM, Franco I, Golding LR: A strategy for cost containment in coronary surgery. JAMA 250:63–66, 1983.
53. Egdahl RH: Cost containment and coronary artery surgery [editorial]. JAMA 250:76–77, 1983.
54. Vander Salm TJ, Blair SA: Effect of reduction of postoperative days in the intensive care unit after coronary artery bypass. J Thorac Cardiovasc Surg 88:558–561, 1984.
55. Moloney TW, Rogers DE: Medical technology: a different view of the contentious debate over costs. N Engl J Med 301:1413–1419, 1979.
56. Foote GA, Schabel SI, Hodges M: Pulmonary complications of the flow-directed balloon-tipped catheter. N Engl J Med 290:927–931, 1974.
57. Wiedemann HP, Matthay MA, Matthay RA: Cardiovascular–pulmonary monitoring in the intensive care unit (part 2). Chest 85:656–668, 1984.
58. Hoar PF, Wilson RM, Mangano DT, Avery II GJ, Szarnicki RJ, Hill JD: Heparin bonding reduces thrombogenicity of pulmonary-artery catheters. N Engl J Med 305:993–995, 1981.
59. Rowley KM, Clubb KS, Walker Smith GJ, Cabin HS: Right-sided infective endocarditis as a consequence of flow-directed pulmonary-artery catheterization: a clinicopathological study of 55 autopsied patients. N Engl J Med 311:1152–1156, 1984.
60. Johnston WE, Royster RL, Choplin RH, Howard G, Mills SA, Tucker WY: Pulmonary artery catheter migration during cardiac surgery. Anesthesiology 64:258–262, 1986.
61. Hardy JF, Morissette M, Taillefer J, Vauclair R: Pathophysiology of rupture of the pulmonary artery by pulmonary artery balloon-tipped catheters. Anesth Analg 62:925–930, 1983.
62. Shah KB, Rao TLK, Laughlin S, El-Etr AA: A review of pulmonary artery catheterization in 6,245 patients. Anesthesiology 61:271–275, 1984.
63. Boyd KD, Thomas SJ, Gold J, Boyd AD: A prospective study of complications of pulmonary artery catheterizations in 500 consecutive patients. Chest 84:245–249, 1983.

8. ROUTINE INSERTION OF PULMONARY ARTERY CATHETERS IS NOT NECESSARY IN ALL PATIENTS UNDERGOING CORONARY ARTERY BYPASS GRAFTING

PHILLIP N. FYMAN
LAWRENCE KUSHINS

PULMONARY ARTERY CATHETERS SHOULD NOT BE INSERTED ROUTINELY FOR PATIENTS UNDERGOING CABG

The debate continues as to whether pulmonary artery (PA) catheters should be routinely used in patients undergoing elective coronary artery bypass grafting (CABG) surgery. We feel that PA catheters should be used only selectively in patients undergoing routine CABG, although there are certain subsets of patients who would benefit, i.e., those with ventricular dysfunction or abnormal wall motion. Generally speaking, the risks of PA catheters outweigh the value of the information gained and should not be used as part of the "CABG protocol."

This is especially true when one considers that there are alternative methods that can be used to obtain the same, if not more precise, information regarding cardiovascular status. In order to support our position, we provide data and information pertaining to four major areas: the pressure obtained from a PA catheter is not exactly what we want and there are safer, alternative methods to obtain this information; the complication rate is not so low that it can be ignored and some of these problems can be lethal; newer techniques provide more sensitive information at much less of a risk; and the cost must be considered.

The balloon flotation thermodilution PA catheter has been used as a monitor during coronary artery bypass surgery since the early 1970s. It has certainly made it simple to measure cardiac output (CO). However, there are significant controversies regarding the degree of correlation between central venous pres-

129

sure (CVP) and pulmonary capillary wedge pressure (PCWP) measurements, between PCWP and left atrial pressure (LAP) or left ventricular end-diastolic volume (LVEDV) measurements, and the utility of the catheter to detect myocardial ischemia. The need for an accurate filling pressure to estimate preload both before and after cardiopulmonary bypass in an effort to determine appropriate therapy for low CO states is obvious, but the question remains as to which filling pressure one should choose.

It has been observed that the CVP correlates well with the PCWP in certain patients. Mangano studied 30 patients undergoing CABG surgery [1]. He compared the relationship of CVP to PCWP at frequent perioperative points in order to determine the degree of correlation between the two methods. He found that the 15 patients with ejection fraction greater than 0.50 and no areas of dyssynergy on preoperative angiocardiography had good correlation of CVP and PCWP over a wide range of pressures. None of these patients had a history of congestive heart failure preoperatively, and none required perioperative inotropic support. Greater than 96% of the data points from these patients allowed a normal CVP to predict a normal PCWP, or an elevated CVP to predict an elevated PCWP. In the one patient in this group who sustained a perioperative myocardial infarction, large changes in PCWP were not estimated well by the CVP.

In each of the 15 patients whose ejection fraction was less than 0.40 or who had left ventricular dyssynergy, there was a poor correlation between the CVP and PCWP. Central venous pressure predicted normal or abnormal PCWP for less than 62% of their data points. Interestingly, for all 15 patients, there was poor correlation prior to bypass, but the correlation improved markedly for six patients immediately after bypass or in the intensive care unit. In those six patients, right ventricular dysfunction occurred, matching the coexisting left ventricular dysfunction, thereby improving the correlation between CVP and PCWP. Although more patients going to surgery today should be medical failures regarding pharmacologic therapy of myocardial ischemia, it does not necessarily follow that they will have low ejection fraction or areas of ventricular dyssynergy. Thus, it can not be assumed that these patients have poor ventricular function.

It has been well documented that right atrial pressure correlated poorly with LAP in patients undergoing valve replacement [2]. However, there is a strong correlation between LAP and PCWP [3], making this an acceptable alternative to PA catheters. Correlation was not as good during tachycardia (due to insufficient time for pressure equalization across the pulmonary vascular bed) or in the presence of increased pulmonary vascular resistance (PVR).

While it is ideal to optimize CO by manipulation of preload following weaning from cardiopulmonary bypass, one must measure left-heart filling pressure in lieu of left ventricular volume or fiber length which in reality is preload. Ellis et al. [4] derived LVEDV from ejection fraction (measured with a coaxial cardiac scintillation probe and serial radiocardiograms) and stroke volume determined by thermodilution. Significant changes (50% increases) in LVEDV occurred with no change in PCWP, while the latter was in the normal 9- to 10-mmHg range. Thus, PCWP did not correlate well with LVEDV, which is what we really want to know.

The PCWP was found to be a poor indicator of LVEDV before or after cardiopulmonary bypass. It is possible that opening the pericardium may alter the pressure–volume relationship, and that the alteration persists postoperatively since the pericardium is left open [5]. It has been reported that raising PCWP following cardiopulmonary bypass while attempting to increase CO, a common practice clinically, may markedly increase LVEDV, altering subendocardial blood flow leading to subendocardial ischemia [4].

A previous study [6] had observed strong correlations between pulmonary artery end-diastolic pressure and LAP at lower pressures, and explained the poorer correlations at higher pressures by variations in pulmonary venous and pulmonary arterial compliances resulting in uneven transmission of pressure waves across the pulmonary vasculature bed. Hardy et al. [7] suggested that the balloon of the PA catheter failed to occlude the pulmonary artery completely at higher pressures, resulting in some communication of proximal pulmonary artery to wedge pressure. This produced strong correlation of PCWP and LAP, but PCWP frequently exceeded LAP.

Mammana et al. [8] compared PCWP and LAP before and after cardiopulmonary bypass and for 16 hours postoperatively. They found significant discrepancies in the early postoperative period and at 4, 8, and 12 h postoperatively, with great individual variation. They suggested that another factor leading to the unpredictably scattered relationship between PCWP and LAP may be mechanical pulmonary venoconstriction. This results from increased pulmonary interstitial water that is caused by hemodilution, which is routinely employed during cardiopulmonary bypass. They also surmised that the use of sodium nitroprusside may exaggerate the left-heart–right-heart disparity by rapidly directly "unloading" the systemic vasculature, while the pulmonary vasculature is "unloaded" more slowly by a time-dependent water diuresis.

Hansen et al. [9] studied 12 patients hourly for 4 h following CABG surgery and ten nonsurgical patients with chronic heart failure to determine whether the PCWP accurately reflected left ventricular preload. They determined left ventricular end-diastolic volume index (LVEDVI) from ejection fraction measured by gated blood pool scintigraphy, and stroke volume calculated from thermodilution CO and heart rate.

In the postoperative patients, changes in PCWP (range 4–32 mmHg) correlated poorly with changes in LVEDVI (range 25–119 ml/m^2), while PCWP and left ventricular stroke work index (LVSWI) also correlated poorly. LVEDVI and LVSWI correlated well. In contrast, the nonsurgical patients had a significant correlation between changes in PCWP and LVEDVI.

The authors explained the discrepancy between PCWP and LVEDVI by acute changes in left ventricular (LV) compliance. They do not believe that this is the result of the rewarming phase of cardiopulmonary bypass, during which such compliance changes have been previously reported [10] since, in the study by Hansen et al., the rewarming phase was over and there were no differences between their earlier and later measurements. Other possible causes of change in ventricular compliance include afterload reduction, use of vasopressors, ventricular interaction, and myocardial ischemia. Changes in LV compliance did not coincide with alterations in PVR or systemic vascular resistance (SVR). Ventricular interaction should not play a significant role here since the pericardium was left open. Transient myocardial ischemia may alter pressure–volume relationships, but was not documented in this study.

Therefore, although it seems best to titrate volume infusion and manipulate hemodynamics by measured left-heart filling pressures and CO, and calculated SVR, significant error may be introduced by assuming that PCWP correlates with LAP and LVEDV. If postoperative care requires estimation of LVEDP, then measuring LAP seems to be the most accurate method.

Systemic vascular resistance calculation is an important parameter to follow and requires measurement of CO among other things. However, CO can be obtained without a PA catheter. Dye dilution CO determination [11] involves injection of indocyanine green into the venous circulation, and withdrawal of blood from the peripheral arterial catheter through a densitometer that measures the change in optical density of the blood at a wavelength of 805 am. This dye is nontoxic and measurements can be repeated every 2 min, since the liver rapidly removes it from the circulation. Computers are available to do the cumbersome calculations. Noninvasive measurement of CO by Doppler probe applied externally or in the esophagus may provide a reliable, accurate method that could be used throughout the perioperative period. It has been shown that Doppler CO correlates well with thermodilution CO during general anesthesia [12].

The use of the PA catheter as a detector of myocardial ischemia is based on observations that, during episodes of angina pectoris, monitored patients often had hemodynamic alterations that included elevation of LVEDP [13]. Kaplan and Wells [14] studied 40 patients undergoing elective myocardial revascularization, and defined myocardial ischemia as ST segment depression > 1 mm, or PCWP trace AC wave > 15 mmHg or V wave > 20 mmHg. Of the 18 patients in whom ischemia was detected, only eight had electrocardiographic (ECG) changes, and three of those had no PCWP trace changes. The remaining ten only had PCWP trace changes. The presumption that the latter patients were experiencing myocardial ischemia is possible, but without corroboration. They suggest in their discussion that the elevation of LVEDP could be associated with subendocardial ischemia as a cause rather than a sign. Of note is the fact that CVP also increased at the same time that the PCWP abnormalities were noted. Since one cannot continuously observe the PCWP trace, one must depend on changes in pulmonary artery pressure to indicate when to look for PCWP trace abnormalities. Therefore, the observer might just as easily observe the CVP trace continuously, and aggressively treat elevations of CVP as a harbinger of ischemia.

Waller et al. [15] attempted to study the use of the information derived from PA catheters by "blinding" the experienced anesthesiologist from the PCWP trace, CO measurements, and SVR calculations. They defined "severe abnormalities" as PCWP > 20 mmHg, PCWP "V" waves > 25 mmHg, cardiac index < 1.5 L/min/m^2, and SVR > 2,500 dyn·s·cm^{-5}. Severe abnormalities were reported in eight of 15 patients, and the anesthesiologists were unaware of these 65% (18 of 28) at the time. Unfortunately we are not informed which abnormalities were detected, nor whether the anesthesiologists interpreted CVP elevation as a sign of ischemia. If the severe abnormalities were mostly low cardiac index or high SVR, we have already discussed obtaining this information without a pulmonary artery catheter. Since the anesthesiologist was informed when severe abnormalities occured, we have no idea what might have happened had they not been told.

In an effort to look at outcome resulting from the failure to use this controversial monitor, Bashein et al. [16] studied patients undergoing elective CABG. They had good LV function defined as ejection fraction greater than 0.40, no history of congestive heart failure, and normal blood pressure response to exercise testing. Of the patients monitored with CVP, 4.7% had PA catheters inserted postoperatively for hemodynamic instability, postoperative hemorrhage, perioperative myocardial infarction, coronary artery spasm, respiratory distress syndrome, or unstated reasons. The in-hospital mortality rate in the study group was only 0.072%, including one death each from: intractable dysrhythmias and pump failure after weaning from cardiopulmonary bypass, anaphylactoid reaction to protamine, sudden postoperative ventricular fibrillation, postoperative hypovolemic shock, and postoperative pneumonia and sepsis in a patient who had had a massive perioperative myocardial infarction. The study patients were not "low risk" despite their normal LV function, since the vast majority had three or more grafts, and 17.3% of patients had left main coronary artery stenosis. The information from this study suggests that only one of 21 patients required insertion of a PA catheter for management of postoperative problems. If this had been done routinely in all patients, the vast majority would have been exposed to the risk of very serious complications without having benefited from the gaining of data that would have improved their outcome.

Data from this study clearly support the concept that patients can undergo CABG safely without PA catheters. It should also be noted that there have been no prospective randomized studies to date demonstrating that PA catheterization and the data obtained from it improve outcome [17]. The question that follows then is: if outcome of surgery is not improved, then why expose the patient to the risk of pulmonary artery complications?

COMPLICATIONS ASSOCIATED WITH PULMONARY ARTERY CATHETERS

Complications associated with PA catheters are relatively rare. However, since they can be catastrophic, i.e., PA hemorrhage, death, etc., they are a real consideration in weighing the balance as to whether placement of a PA catheter should be done.

When the catheter is inserted percutaneously, accidental arterial cannulation can occur. While this is possible when inserting a CVP line, the consequences can be much more severe with a PA catheter because of the larger bore introducer. The sequelae that arise from traumatizing an artery include disruption of an atheromatous plaque, causing embolization of debris or dissection of the vessel. In either case, impairment of blood flow results, leading to ischemia in that vascular distribution. Even after proper placement of the catheter, venous thrombosis of a major vessel can develop [18–20].

Arrhythmias are frequently associated with insertion of PA catheters. Although usually transient, there arrhythmias are life-threatening. In one prospective study, it was found that 90 out of 116 intensive care unit (ICU) patients developed arrhythmias during PA catheter insertion [20]; 53 patients developed premature ventricular contractions and an alarming 27 patients experienced short runs of ventricular tachycardia. A transient right bundle branch block developed in three patients. In another study done on ICU patients, one patient developed intractable ventricular tachycardia and could not be resuscitated [21]. The lower incidence of ventricular arrhythmias—10% in this study compared to 78% in the former study—can probably be explained by different methods used to detect arrhythmias. When the cardiac rhythm was recorded continuously as opposed to observation only, the incidence of arrhythmias was usually higher.

A PA catheter-induced fatal arrhythmia also occurred in another study [22] where 40 critically ill patients had their ECG recorded; 68% experienced ventricular ectopy; 48% [19] developed ventricular tachycardia, which was sustained in three patients; and ventricular fibrillation occurred in one patient who could not be resuscitated.

Attempts to decrease the incidence of ventricular irritability have been made by administering prophylactic lidocaine [23]. However, this was found to be ineffective. The control group experienced ventricular ectopy 65% of the time while the lidocaine-treated group had a peak incidence of 76%. Ventricular tachycardia occurred in 19% of patients in the control group compared to 13% of the patients who received lidocaine 2 mg/kg.

In another study prospectively evaluating PA catheter-associated complications, 72% were observed to have ventricular ectopy [24]. In 3%, the premature ventricular contractions were persistent and required intravenous lidocaine for suppression. One patient with a preexisting left bundle branch block developed complete heart block and pacing was needed.

Pulmonary infarction and/or hemorrhage are other potentially life-threatening complications associated with PA catheters. Although perforation of the pulmonary artery by a PA catheter is rare, it can lead to a fatal outcome. In one series of five patients with pulmonary hemorrhage, four expired [25]. This problem is of major concern when dealing with patients at increased risk for this complication, i.e., those who will be anticoagulated for cardiopulmonary bypass, in patients with preexisting pulmonary hypertension, and in situations when the catheter may migrate distally [26]. During cardiopulmonary bypass, distal migration of the catheter can occur for a number of reasons, i.e., catheter stiffening with hypothermia, excessive slack of the catheter in the right ventricle, and manipulation of the ehart during cardiac surgery. Because the complications associated with distal catheter migration can be so catastrophic, there have been recommendations to withdraw the catheter into the right ventricle during cardiopulmonary bypass [27].

The various therapeutic modalities that are avilable if hemorrhage should occur, such as positive end-expiratory pressure [28, 29] and maintaining the position of the catheter with the balloon inflated, are not always effective in preventing a fatality. This emphasizes the fact that prevention is more effective than treatment, and insertion of a PA catheter can result in serious sequelae without effective treatment.

Pulmonary artery catheterization has been associated with causing lesions of the right side of the heart. In one study of 142 consecutive autopsies, there were 55 patients who had PA catheters inserted antermortem [30]: 29 patients (53%) had right-sided endocardial lesions compared to only three (3%) of 87 patients who did not have intracardiac catheters inserted; 56% of the lesions were located on the pulmonic valve, and an almost equal distribution (10%–15%) on the tricuspid valve, right artium, and right ventricle, with 5% in the pulmonary trunk. Approximately two-thirds of the lesions were thrombi and one-third were subendocardial hemorrhages. Eight of the 26 thrombi were found to be infected. Positive blood cultures were obtained in 11 of 55 catheterized patients and four of these developed right-sided endocarditis. None of the 87 patients who were not catheterized had evidence at autopsy of infective endocarditis. It should be noted that these investigators found no correlation between right-sided cardiac lesions and duration of time catheter was in place, site of catheter insertion, pulmonary artery pressures, or the size of the right ventricle. This makes it difficult, if not impossible, to predict who is at risk for these complications. This higher incidence of right-sided lesions in patients with PA catheters corraborates earlier findings. In a previous study, 61% of catheterized hearts examined were found to have mural thrombi [31]. Other pathologic lesions found included valvular hemorrhage (31%) and aseptic valvular lesions (14%). These lesions are usually not found in these locations, strongly suggesting that they were catheter induced.

Pulmonary valve injury and insufficiency have also been reported in patients who have undergone right-heart catheterization [20, 32]. Although rare, this occurrence can be life threatening. It is postulated that the constant motion of the heart against the catheter can lead to endothelial damage, resulting in valvular dysfunction. Pulmonary artery catheter-induced tricuspid valve damage has also been reported [33].

Another rare, but extremely serious, complication of PA catheterization is intracardiac knotting [34, 35]. This usually occurs when an excessive length of the catheter has been inserted into the right ventricle, permitting it to coil around itself, forming a knot. The situation can be further worsened by intertwining with the chordae tendinae or papillary muscle and interfering with valvular function when attempts to withdraw the catheter are made. In extreme circumstances, open-heart surgery may be required to remove the catheter.

This discussion of PA catheter-associated complications emphasizes the complexity of this procedure. Because of the possibility for life-threatening sequelae developing, this should not be done as a shotgun approach to everyone undergoing CABG, especially in view of the fact that it has not been shown to improve outcome.

AN ALTERNATIVE METHOD FOR EVALUATING CARDIAC FUNCTION

While PA catheterization is a common intraoperative method to monitor cardiovascular status, alternative methods are available. These provide reliable, reproducible data without many, if not all, of the risks associated with a PA catheter.

One alternative to PA catheterization is transesophageal echocardiography (TEE). Since its introduction in 1954, up until the present, thoracic ultrasound has been an important diagnostic tool in clinical cardiology. It has the capabilities of fast and accurate evaluation of valvular anatomy and function. Cardiac ultra-sound can also assess ventricular function.

Although transthoracic echocardiography provides valuable information regarding cardiac function, there are a number of factors that limit its usefulness during the intraoperative and immediate postoperative periods. During cardiac surgery, its location would interfere with the procedure; postoperatively, dressing and changes in the chest wall also would impair its usefulness.

In order to circumvent many of these obstacles, transesophageal echocardiography has been developed. The instrument consists of a phased-array or M-mode transducer fixed to the tip of a commercially available gastroscope [36–38]. It is simple to introduce and position in the esophagus [39]. There is minimal discomfort, it can be done easily in the awake as well as the anesthetized patient, and it is a skill that is relatively easy to master. Another advantage of TEE is that its use is associated with minimal, if any, risks or complications.

Early studies have demonstrated that there is good correlation between data obtained by transthoracic echocardiograms and TEE [36, 39, 40]. One group of investigators found that there was a high degree of correlation between the two methods when evaluating the aortic valve, left atrium, and mitral valve [39]. However, the correlation was much weaker for aortic root measurements.

Left ventricular function was not measured due to technical difficulties, although later investigators did confirm the ability of TEE to assess LV function [36, 40]. Calculation of cardiac output by TEE has also been shown to correlate well with the more invasive methods [40, 41].

One of the major advantages of echocardiography is that it provides continuous and sensitive information regarding segmental ventricular wall motion. If abnormalities are diagnosed and treated early enough, irreversible damage may be avoided. When a PA catheter is used to monitor ventricular function, abnormalities may manifest themselves only later, when global ischemia has occurred. In one study, a dog model was used to determine how sensitive and specific echocardiography is in detecting ischemia-induced abnormal ventricular wall mation [42]. The standard used for comparison, which is the accepted gold standard, was wall motion assessed by sonomicrometers implanted in the LV wall. The echocardiographic transducer was placed directly on the pericardium. This study confirmed that echocardiography is a sensitive and specific technique to detect segmental wall abnormalities related to transient ischemia. Whenever there were ischemic changes detected by sonomicrometry, they were present on echocardiogram. When wall motion was normal as evaluated by sonomicrometry, it was normal on echocardiogram. The sensitivity of TEE for detecting ventricular wall motion abnormalities and deterioration of cardiac function intraoperatively has also been demonstrated in humans [43]. A group of 25 patients undergoing aortic reconstructive surgery was evaluated. All of these patients had PA catheters inserted for cardiac monitoring as well as transesophageal echocardiograms. During cross-clamping of the aorta above the celiac artery, systemic and pulmonary artery pressures were maintained within the normal range. However, transesophageal echocardiography detected distinct abnormalities of LV function. These consisted of increases in LV end-systolic and end-diastolic areas, wall motion abnormalities, and a reduction in ejection fraction. This indicates that TEE has the capacity to be more sensitive in detecting early myocardial dysfunction then the PA catheter and permits earlier treatment.

Another advantage of TEE over PA catheterization is that continuous information is obtained. With a PA catheter, two of the most important parameters that we measure, cardiac output and pulmonary artery wedge pressure, can only be obtained intermittently, which can result in a decrease in response time from cardiovascular deterioration to therapeutic intervention, increasing the risk of cardiovascular morbidity or mortality.

One application of TEE, which has not been investigated fully, is the detection of intracardiac air bubbles. If it is found that TEE is a useful diagnostic tool in this respect, it would certainly minimize the potential for air emboli in cardiac procedures where a chamber of the heart is entered. In this regard, echocardiography would be more sensitive and specific than a PA catheter, where an elevated pressure can mean any number of things.

In summary, TEE provides more sensitive information on a continuous basis regarding the cardiovascular system than a PA catheter. In addition, the risk of untoward events resulting from the monitoring device is much less. We submit that TEE compares favorably to the more traditional PA catheter as a monitor of cardiac function. Furthermore, the technology has been developed to the extent that TEE is a clinically useful tool in the operating room. Dye dilution cardiac output is another alternative to PA catheterization. It is economical, simple to perform, and permits calculation of the majority of the information a PA line gives, i.e., SVR, stroke work index, etc., while avoiding the hazards.

ECONOMIC CONSIDERATIONS

The increased cost of a PA catheter compared to a CVP catheter has to be considered when making the decision to use this routinely in all patients undergoing CABG. In today's economic environment, the pressure is toward cost containment. With the cost of medical services placed at $316 billion, or 7.5% of the gross national product, and increasing annually, there are many forces attempting to keep the cost of health care down.

Various approaches have been used to try and achieve this goal with regard to CABG. One group of investigators looked at the expense of cardiac surgery in a community hospital [44]. They discussed with each department the costs that they incurred, and attempted to get them to evaluate how necessary those tests or procedures were. Routine procedures and therapies that were eliminated included postoperative IPPB therapy and "high"-dose steroids. This led to an 11% reduction in the cost of hospitalization. Another strategy to reduce the cost of CABG was to admit the patient the morning of surgery [45]. In this study, the cost of this procedure was reduced by 1%. This resulted, among other things, from a decrease in the length of stay and PA catheterization was not done routinely. Other investigators have evaluated the economic impact of reducing postoperative ICU days from two to one [46]. Although total cost was not significantly decreased statistically, there was a significant decrease in room costs and amount spent on arterial blood gases. There was no difference in complication rate between groups and no deaths occurred in either group.

The cost of PA catheterization can be broken down as follows. Catheter cost varies from $80 to $150; transducers (disposable) and pressure tubing cost ~$20. Physicians' fees for insertion range from $250 to $500; other factors that must be considered, but are difficult to place a dollar value on, are the monitors that must be used and possibly more intensive nursing care and longer ICU stays. Based on these assumptions, the cost of PA catheterization will be ~$400–$750. If this is not done routinely, the cost of an uncomplicated CABG (~$20,000) can be reduced by 2%–4%. It should be noted that this estimate may be high for a couple of reasons. It makes the assumption that no patient undergoing a CABG will receive a PA catheter, which is not true. As we stated at the onset, there are some subsets of patients who clearly benefit from it. Furthermore, it does not factor in the cost of a CVP, which almost all other patients will have inserted. However, the cost of this is much less. On the other hand, complications leading to longer hospitalizations or other therapies, such as chest tubes, were not included in this estimate. This may tend to offset the factors mentioned above that underestimate the savings. Although a savings of 2%–4% of the total cost may appear to be only a minor savings, because of the large volume of cases done nationwide approaching 200,000 annually, we are dealing with a large dollar amount. Furthermore, if a 2% savings can be realized with this approach, and an 11% savings and a 10% savings can be achieved with the strategies noted above, these begin to add up to an appreciable reduction in cost. Put in this context, the cost of inserting a PA catheter selectively in only certain patients undergoing CABG can lead to a significant reduction in cost of this procedure on a national basis.

In conclusion, we feel that routine insertion of a PA catheter in all patients undergoing CABG is not warranted. The risk of increased morbidity and mortality, the additional costs, the availability of alternative methods, and the lack of any data that indicate this procedure improves patient outcome all weigh against the recommendation that it be used in each patient having this procedure.

REFERENCES

1. Mangano DT: Monitoring pulmonary arterial pressure in coronary artery disease. Anesthesiology 53:364–370, 1980.
2. Sarin CL, Yalav E, Clement AJ, Braimbridge MV: The necessity for measurement of left atrial pressure after cardiac valve surgery. Thorax 25:185–189, 1970.
3. Lappas D, Lell WA, Gabel JC, et al.: Indirect measurements of left-atrial pressure in surgical patients: pulmonary-capillary wedge and pulmonary-artery diastolic pressures compared with left-atrial pressure. Anesthesiology 38:394–397, 1973.
4. Ellis RJ, Mangano DT, Van Dyke DC: Relationship of wedge pressure to end-diastolic volume in patients undergoing myocardial revascularization. J Thorac Cardiovasc Surg 78:605–613, 1979.
5. Glantz SA, Parwley WW, Tyberg JV: The pericardium substantially affects the left ventricular diastolic pressure–volume relationship in the dog. Circ Res 42:433–441, 1978.
6. Falicov RE, Resnekow L: Relationship of the pulmonary end-diastolic pressure to the left ventricular end-diastolic and mean filling pressures in patients with and without left ventricular dysfunction. Circulation 42:65–73, 1970.
7. Hardy JD, Carcia JB, Hardy JA, Harkins MH: Fluid replacement monitoring. Ann Surg 180:162–166, 1974.
8. Mammana RB, Hiro S, Levitsky S, et al.: Inaccuracy of pulmonary capillary wedge pressure when compared to left atrial pressure in the early postsurgical period. J Thorac Cardiovasc Surg 84:420–425, 1982.
9. Hansen RM, Viquerat CE, Matthau MA, et al.: Poor correlation between pulmonary arterial wedge pressure and left ventricular end-diastolic volume after coronary artery bypass graft surgery. Anesthesiology 64:764–770, 1986.
10. Ivanon J, Weisel RD, Mickelborough LL, et al.: Rewarming hypovolemia after aortocoronary artery bypass surgery. Crit Care Med 12:1049–1054, 1984.
11. Prys-Roberts C: The measurement of cardiac output. Br J Anaesth 41:751–60, 1969.
12. Kumar A, Minagoe S, Thangathurai D, et al.: Non-invasive measurement of cardiac output during general anesthesia by continuous wave Doppler esophageal probe: comparison with simultaneous thermodilution cardiac output. Anesthesiology 63:A68, 1985.

13. Wiener L, Dwyer EM, Cox JM: Left ventricular hemodynamics in exercise induced angina pectoris. Circulation 38:240–249, 1968.
14. Kaplan JA, Wells PH: Early diagnosis of myocardial ischemia using the pulmonary arterial catheter. Anesth Analg 60:789–793, 1981.
15. Waller JL, Johnson SP, Kaplan JA: Usefulness of pulmonary artery catheters during aortocoronary bypass surgery [abstr]. Anesth Analg 61:221–222, 1982.
16. Bashein G, Johnson PW, David KB, Ivey TD: Elective coronary bypass surgery without pulmonary artery catheter monitoring. Anesthesiology 63:451–454, 1985.
17. Keefer KR, Barash PC: Pulmonary artery catheterization: a decade of clinical progress? Chest 84:241–242, 1983.
18. Dye LE, Segall PH, Russell RO, et al.: Deep venous thrombosis of the upper extremity associated with the use of the Swan–Ganz catheter. Chest 73:673–675, 1978.
19. Yona FH, Oblath R, Jaffe H, et al.: Massive thrombosis associated with the use of the Swan–Ganz catheter. Chest 65:682–684, 1974.
20. Elliot G, Zimmerman GA, Clemmer GP: Complications of pulmonary artery catheterization in the care of critically ill patients. Chest 76:647–652, 1979.
21. Sise MJ, Hollingsworth P, Brimm JE, et al.: Complications of the flow-directly pulmonary artery catheter. Crit Care Med 9:315–318, 1981.
22. Sprung C, Jacobs L, Carallis P, et al.: hazards of PA catheter [letter]. N Engl J Med 302:807, 1980.
23. Salmenplia M, Peltola K, Rosenberg P: Does prophylactic lidocaine control cardiac arrythmias associated with pulmonary artery catheterization? Anesthesiology 56:210–212, 1982.
24. Shah RB, Rao TL, Laughlin S, et al.: A review of pulmonary artery catheterization in 6,245 patients. Anesthesiology 61:271–275, 1984.
25. Pape LA, Haffajie LI, Markis JE, et al.: Fatal pulmonary artery hemorrhage after use of the flow-directed balloon-tipped catheter. Ann Intern Med 90:344–347, 1979.
26. Johnston WE, Royster RL, Choplin RH, et al.: Pulmonary artery catheter migration during cardiac surgery. Anesthesiology 64:258–262, 1986.
27. Stone GJ, Khambatta HJ, McDaniel D: Cardiopulmonary bypass and catheter induced pulmonary-artery hemorrhage. In: Proceedings abstracts of the fifth annual meeting of the Society of Cardiovascular Anesthesiologist, 1982, pp 199–200.
28. Rice RL, Pifane R, El-Etr A, et al.: Management of endobronchial hemorrhage during cardiopulmonary bypass. J Thorac Cardiovas Surg 81:800–8001, 1981.
29. Scuderi PE, Prough DS, Price JD, et al.: Lessation of pulmonary artery catheter induced endobronchial hemorrhage associated with the use of PEEP. Anesth Analg 62:236–238, 1983.
30. Rowley KM, Clubb KS, Smith GJ, et al.: Right sided infective endocarditis as a consequence of flow-directed pulmonary artery catheterization. N Engl J Med 311:1152–1156, 1984.
31. Lange HW, Galliani CA, Edwards JE: Local complications associated with indwelling Swan–Ganz catheters: autopsy study of 36 cases. Am J Cardiol 52:1108–1111, 1983.
32. O'Toole JD, Wurtzbacher JJ, Wearner NE, et al.: Pulmonary valve injury and insufficiency during pulmonary artery catheterization. N Engl J Med 301:1167–1168, 1979.
33. Boscoe MJ, de Lange S: Damage to the tricuspid valve with Swan–Ganz catheter. Br Med J 283:346–347, 1981.
34. Lipp H, O'Donoghue K, Resnekov L: Intracardiac knotting of a flow directed balloon catheter [letter]. N Engl J Med 284:220, 1971.
35. Fibrich EE, Tuohy GF: Intracardiac knotting of a flow-directed balloon-typed catheter. Anesth Analg 59:217–219, 1980.
36. Schwartz L, Cahalan MK, Gutman J, et al.: Intraoperative monitoring of left ventricular performance by transesophageal M-mode and 2-D echocardiograph. Am J Cardiol 49:956, 1982.
37. Schluter M, Hinricks A, Thier W, et al.: Transesophageal two-dimensional echocardiography: comparison of ultrasonic and anatomic sections. Am J Cardiol 53:1173–1178, 1984.
38. Schluter M, Langenstein BA, Plster J, et al.: Transesophageal cross sectional echocardiography with a phased array transducer system. Br Heart J 48:67–72, 1982.
39. Frazin L, Talano JV, Steplanides L, et al.: Esophageal echocardiography. Circulation 54: 102–108, 1976.
40. Matsumoto M, Oka Y, Strom J, et al.: Application of transesophageal echocardiography to continuous intraoperative monitoring of left ventricular performance. Am J Cardiol 46:95–105, 1980.

41. Matsumoto M, Oka Y, Lin YT, et al.: Transesophageal echocardiography. NY State J Med 79:19–21, 1979.
42. Pandian N, Kerber RE: Two dimensional echocardiography in experimental coronary stenosis. Circulation 66:597–602, 1982.
43. Roizen MF, Beaupre PN, Alpert RA, et al.: Monitoring with two-dimensional transesophageal echocardiography. J Vasc Surg 1:300–305, 1984.
44. Tomatis LA, Schlosser RJ, Diaki M, et al.: Cost containment via expense rationalization in open heart surgery. J Thorac Cardiovasc Surg 77:448–451, 1979.
45. Loop FD, Christiansen EK, Lester JL, et al.: A strategy for cost containment in coronary surgery. JAMA 250:63–66, 1983.
46. Vander Salm T, Blair S: Effect of reduction of postoperative days in the intensive care unit after coronary artery bypass. J Thorac Cardiovasc Surg 88:558–561, 1984.

9. GENERAL ANESTHESIA IS PREFERABLE FOR PATIENTS UNDERGOING CAROTID ENDARTERECTOMY

CAROL L. LAKE

Carotid endarterectomy presents the anesthesiologist with three major problems: maintenance of oxygenation to the brain during the temporary, but critical, period of occlusion of the common, internal, and external carotid arteries; dislodgement of emboli from atheromatous plaques during arterial manipulation; and, finally, reperfusion injury to the brain when the carotid clamp is released. The brain has a high metabolic rate for oxygen (CMR_{O_2}) of ~3 ml/min/100 g brain, with little storage capacity for oxygen. The oxygen content of blood passing through the brain decreases from 19 to 21 ml/dl. Glucose is the major source of energy. Since the initial procedure by Carrea et al. [1] in 1951, anesthesiologists and surgeons have sought ways to prevent neurologic deficits resulting from even brief periods of inadequate cerebral perfusion. The administration of general anesthesia obviates many of the problems posed by carotid endarterectomy. Oxygenation, airway, blood pressure, and cerebral metabolism are effectively controlled.

PATHOPHYSIOLOGY AND INDICATIONS FOR SURGERY

If the circle of Willis is patent, major occlusion of both carotid and vertebral arteries bilaterally must be present before cerebral blood flow decreases. Less severe lesions may cause symptoms of transient or permanent ischemia. A transient ischemic attack (TIA) is an episode of focal neurologic dysfunction or generalized cerebral ischemia lasting minutes to hours, but with complete resolution within 24 h [2]. TIA often presents with weakness of the face or upper extremity, but occasionally monocular blindness (amaurosis fugax), sensory abnormalities, hypertension, or cardiac dysrhythmias occur [3]. Reversible ischemic neurologic deficits with TIA, with or without residual

143

Table 9-1. Indications for carotid endarterectomy

Transient ischemic attack (TIA)
Asymptomatic carotid stenosis
Reversible ischemic neurologic deficit
Central retinal artery occlusion
Completed strokes
? Stroke in evolution

neurologic deficit, particularly if the TIAs are increasing in frequency or severity [4], and to asymptomatic patients with identifiable arteriosclerotic plaques occluding more than 50% of the lumen of the vessel, or contralateral lesions occluding more than 80% of the vessel lumen [5]. Carotid endarterectomy for stroke in evolution results in substantially improved quality of life over that of medically treated controls [4]. Colgan et al. [6] and Quinones-Baldrich and Moore [7] have questioned the wisdom of prophylactic endarterectomy in asymptomatic carotid stenosis as the cumulative stroke-free interval over 3 years is 97%, which is similar to the morbidity/mortality data for carotid endarterectomy. The morbidity and mortality from intervention may be greater than indicated by observation alone [8]. Patients with asymptomatic lesions should, however, be instructed to return immediately if symptoms develop. Endarterectomy is also indicated in patients with reversible ischemic neurologic deficits with negative CAT scans and angiographically demonstrated lesions [9].

Endarterectomy may be performed after recent total occlusion and reestablish flow, but can turn an anemic infarct into a hemorrhagic infarct with subsequent intracerebral hemorrhage [10] with a surgical mortality of 40%–50% [11]. Central retinal artery occlusion associated with carotid lesions is also an indication. Even after completed stable strokes, carotid endarterectomy is protective against new neurologic deficits [12]. Carotid endarterectomy may also be indicated in patients with carotid stenosis undergoing cardiac surgery in which a 14.9% incidence of hemispheric neurologic deficits has been noted [13] (compared to a 5% incidence of neurodeficits without carotid disease) (table 9-1). Medical management of significant carotid stenosis results in a greater incidence of cerebrovascular events or death than with endarterectomy [14]. Carotid endarterectomy is contraindicated in patients with early acute cerebral infarction, stroke in evolution, an occluded internal carotid artery, a tandem siphon lesion more severe than the more distal carotid lesions, or in those with limited life expectancy secondary to other medical problems.

DIAGNOSTIC TECHNIQUES

Significance of bruits on physical examination

Preoperative evaluation of adult patients should include auscultation of the neck. Cervical bruits, encountered in 10% of patients over age 40 years [15], are frequently caused by a stenotic lesion of the internal carotid artery, although bruits from the heart, thyroid, and veins may be present. Although neck bruits are valuable indicators of carotid stenosis, the addition of Doppler ultrasound to auscultation improves the accuracy [16]. However, significant carotid disease can be present in the absence of bruits [17].

Indirect tests

Ophthalmodynamometry (OPD)

A calibrated strain gauge is utilized to apply lateral scleral pressure to produce gradual obliteration of flow in the retinal arteries during continuous ophthalmoscopic observation. The point of complete obliteration is the systolic pressure and that pressure required to produce intermittent collapse, the diastolic pressure. The relative ophthalmic artery pressure difference between the two eyes is determined and should be less than 15% if the carotid circulation is normal. Ophthalmic arterial stenosis may yield false-positive results and bilateral carotid disease may be missed with this technique [18]. False-negative tests occur with extensive collateral circulation and hypertension [19].

Ocular plethysmography (OPG)

Either pneumoplethysmography [20, 21] or fluid-filled oculoplethysmography [22, 23] can localize carotid lesions. Pneumoplethysmography involves the application of a vacuum to the sclera to determine systolic ophthalmic artery pressures as pulsations return on release of the vacuum. Pressures in both eyes are tested as is their relationship to brachial pressure. Inequality of eye pressures with the ratio of ophthalmic–brachial pressure below 0.66 or a combination of an ophthalmic–brachial pressure ratio below 0.6 and equal ophthalmic pressures indicate carotid stenosis [14]. OPG is insensitive to stenoses of less than 60%. Ophthalmic artery stenosis causes false-positive results. However, although a negative OPG does not exclude high-grade stenosis, depending upon compensatory collateral flow, it may indicate its hemodynamic significance [21].

The fluid-filled technique, described by Kartchner et al. [22, 23], evaluates the comparative timing of ocular pulse arrival by pressure transducers in ocular cups held by vacuum on the cornea. There is a relative delay in pulse arrival on the side of an internal carotid stenosis. However, difficulties in the detection of bilateral disease, ulcerated plaques, stenosis of less than 50%, or differentiation of high-grade stenosis from total occlusion may occur [18, 24]. Such periorbital tests as OPD and OPG cannot distinguish between operable and inoperable or totally occluded carotid lesions.

A cerebral hemodynamic test is a noninvasive preoperative or intraoperative evaluation of unilateral or bilateral carotid compression in which the electroencephalogram (EEG), changes in neurologic status, and the photopulses recorded from cutaneous areas supplied by internal and external carotid arteries are monitored [25] to document appropriate head position or other maneuvers to prevent reduced cerebral blood flow.

Direct tests

Sonography

Ultrasonic (Doppler) flowmeters can accurately determine common carotid, internal carotid, and more peripheral arterial blood flow velocities. These devices assess local frequency characteristics of the Doppler signal by either aural or spectral analysis. Doppler technology is more sensitive to high-grade carotid stenosis that it is to lesions of less than 50%. However, it can differentiate stenoses of less than 50% from completely occluded vessels [18]. Carotid flow normally decreases with patient age and the ratio of flow between the two carotid arteries increases in patients with transient ischemic attacks or other intracranial pathology [26].

Ocular flow and the effects of carotid compression upon ocular flow can be determined with bidirectional Doppler. Blood flow in branches of the ophthalmic artery such as the supraorbital artery is normally antegrade, out of the orbit. Flow is augmented by compression of the superficial temporal artery and attenuated by compression of the ipsilateral carotid. In the presence of carotid stenosis, flow is attenuated by external carotid compression (collateral vessel) and may actually become retrograde. These techniques are less sensitive to stenoses of less than 50%, are unable to distinguish ulcerative lesions, and fail to differentiate between high-grade lesions and total occlusion [27].

A duplex carotid sonogram is a real-time B-mode ultrasonic imaging technique coupled with a 5-Hz pulsed Doppler. Pulsed Doppler techniques add depth discrimination to the flow pattern sensed by the device. The sensitivity, accuracy, and specificity of duplex scanning are greater than with either technique individually or with OPG [28]. Duplex scan provides two types of information: an abnormal audible signal and an abnormal reflected spectrum of the Doppler signal. The abnormal audible signal consists of a harsh high-frequency response indicating turbulent high-velocity flow [28]. Abnormal reflected spectra are characterized by spectral broadening with loss of the low-frequency "window" of normal arteries, and by peak frequency of 4 kHz or greater in the reflected signal [28]. A normal vessel has less than a 3.5-Hz peak frequency shift with no spectral broadening. A peak frequency shift of less than 3.5 Hz correlated with less than 30% stenosis in the artery, 3.5–4 Hz with 31–50% stenosis, 4–8 Hz with 80%–90% stenosis, and greater than 8 Hz with greater than 90% stenosis [29, 30] (figure 9-1).

However, evaluation with a pulsed Doppler velocimeter demonstrates that disturbance of the velocity profile occurs before significant changes in volume flow or angiogram occur [31]. Thus, the structural appearance of the arteries may not consistently denote the dynamic flow conditions [31]. In the postoperative state, the Doppler and other ultrasound devices provide more detail

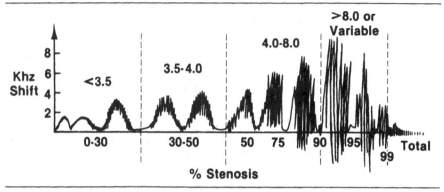

Figure 9-1. Carotid sonogram. From Jacobs N. Metal: Radiology 154:386, 1985 with permission of author and publisher.

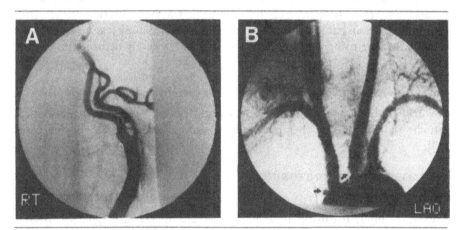

Figure 9-2. Digital subtraction angiogram.

and easier localization of technical problems than does an electromagnetic flowmeter [32].

Carotid angiography

Patients with positive findings on noninvasive testing usually undergo carotid arteriography. Digital subtraction angiography (DSA), a computerized fluoroscopic technique using intravenous radiocontrast, may eventually render retrograde arteriography obsolete (figure 9-2). Pulsed x-rays of 0.05- to 0.1-s duration acquire the images, which are then subjected to either temporal or energy subtraction. Using the temporal subtraction technique, the original image prior to contrast is stored and then compared to images obtained after contrast, but free from the structural background of bone, soft tissue, or other images. Energy subtraction techniques involve acquisition of images using low- and high-energy that can be combined to subtract bone or soft tissue and enhance blood vessels. The intraarterial route for DSA is also being evaluated. Problems with DSA include optimal subtraction techniques in calcified vessles, overlying vessels, poor cardiac output causing long transit time of the intravenous contrast, and patient motion [18].

Conventional transarterial carotid angiography remains the "gold standard" for diagnosis. Either direct carotid puncture or retrograde brachial or transfemoral catheter techniques are used. Biplane views are usually obtained. Arch aortography may be performed concurrently if carotid angiography fails to delineate the cause of cerebrovascular insufficiency. During angiography, a trial of balloon occlusion of a carotic artery can be performed to assess the adequacy of collateral flow in the conscious state [33].

Ivey and colleagues [34] question the need for routine arteriography of asymptomatic patients to document the presence of carotid stenosis prior to cardiac surgery. These investigators noted that asymptomatic patients with high-grade lesions, documented by ultrasound carotid duplex scan, underwent cardiac surgery using extracorporeal circulation without neurologic damage [34].

Interventional revascularization: fibrinolytic therapy and ballon angioplasty

For inaccessible lesions of the internal carotid system occurring acutely, local intraarterial fibrinolytic therapy has been successful in a few reported cases [35].

INTRAOPERATIVE MONITORING

"Stump pressure"

The distal internal carotid back pressure ("stump pressure") is the arterial pressure in the internal carotid distal to clamps on the common and external carotid arteries (figure 9-3). A stump pressure of 50–60 mmHg is often considered the critical level [36] as few patients experience neurologic deficits with stump pressures greater than 50 torr [37]. On the other hand, numerous patients with stump pressure between 30 and 40 torr also fail to suffer neurologic deficits, and the critical stump pressure may be more like 30–35 torr [37]. Unfortunately, no safe stump pressure has been identified that prevents neurologic damage, nor does stump pressure correlate with regional cerebral blood flow, EEG evidence of ischemia, or cerebral tolerance to cross-clamping in all patients [36, 38]. Low stump pressures only roughly correlate with ischemic EEG changes [39]. Induced hypertension and hypocarbia may increase the stump pressure, while hypercarbia has no effect [40, 41]. Stump pressure and regional cerebral blood flow during occlusion are inversely related during halothane, enflurane, or isoflurane anesthesia [38]. The lowest stump pressures and highest cerebral blood flows are seen during halothane anesthesia in patients with cerebral flows greater than 18 ml/100 g/min [36]. The highest stump pressures and lowest cerebral flows are seen during droperidol and fentanyl

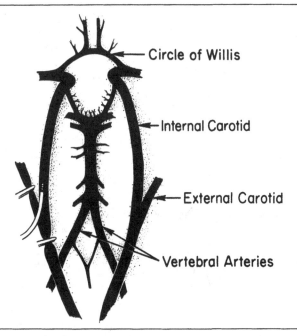

Circle of Willis

Internal Carotid

External Carotid

Vertebral Arteries

Figure 9-3. Measurement of stump pressure. From Lake CL: Cardiovascular Anesthesia. New York: Springer-Verlag, 1985, p. 411 with permission of publisher.

(Innovar) anesthesia. Sublett and colleagues [42] have demonstrated the unreliability of stump pressure to indicate the need for a shunt in patients under regional anaesthesia.

The need to measure not only the back pressure, but also the jugular venous pressure, to determine the difference as an index of the cerebral perfusion pressure was noted by Archie and Feldman [32]. However, cerebral perfusion pressure is also dependent upon intracranial pressure, which was not measured in their series [32]. The refinement of adding the jugular venous pressure may identify more high-risk patients than those noted by low carotid back pressures alone. Measurement of the jugular bulb Po_2 alone indicates the oxygenation of the entire cerebral hemisphere, rather than regional ischemia [43]. Focal areas of ischemia contribute little to the jugular venous pool, making jugular venous saturation a poor guide to cerebral function.

Somatosensory evoked potentials

Despite the expense, technical difficulties, and cumbersome, complicated equipment, somatosensory evoked potentials (SEPs) appear useful as monitors during carotid surgery [44]. They are electrical potentials, recorded from scalp electrodes, generated in response to a specific stimulus, either visual, auditory, or somatosensory. SEPs are abolished at cerebral blood flows of less than 15–20 ml/min [45]. Cerebral ischemia is suggested by reduction in amplitude,

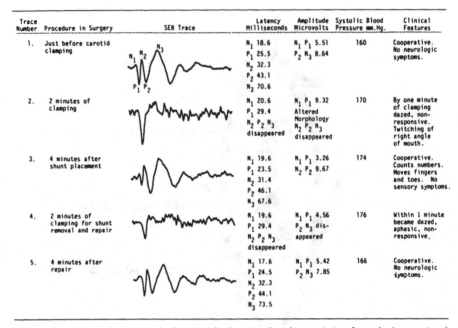

Trace Number	Procedure in Surgery	SER Trace	Latency Milliseconds	Amplitude Microvolts	Systolic Blood Pressure mm.Hg.	Clinical Features
1.	Just before carotid clamping		N_1 18.6 P_1 25.5 N_2 32.3 P_2 43.1 N_3 70.6	N_1 P_1 5.51 P_2 N_3 8.64	160	Cooperative. No neurologic symptoms.
2.	2 minutes of clamping		N_1 20.6 P_1 29.4 N_2 P_2 N_3 disappeared	N_1 P_1 9.32 Altered Morphology N_2 P_2 N_3 disappeared	170	By one minute of clamping dazed, non-responsive. Twitching of right angle of mouth.
3.	4 minutes after shunt placement		N_1 19.6 P_1 23.5 N_2 31.4 P_2 46.1 N_3 67.6	N_1 P_1 3.26 N_2 P_2 9.67	174	Cooperative. Counts numbers. Moves fingers and toes. No sensory symptoms.
4.	2 minutes of clamping for shunt removal and repair		N_1 19.6 P_1 29.4 N_2 P_2 N_3 disappeared	N_1 P_1 4.56 P_2 N_3 disappeared	176	Within 1 minute became dazed, aphasic, non-responsive.
5.	4 minutes after repair		N_1 17.6 P_1 24.5 N_2 32.3 P_2 44.1 N_3 73.5	N_1 P_1 5.42 P_2 N_3 7.85	166	Cooperative. No neurologic symptoms.

Figure 9-4. Somatosensory evoked potentials. Reprinted with permission from the International Anesthesia Research Society from Somatosensory evoked responses during carotid endarterectomy by S.S. Moorthy. Anesthesia Analgesia 61:882, 1982.

waveform distortion, or prolongation of latencies in the SEP [46]. Cerebral ischemia affects the amplitude of the SEP more than its latency. Figure 9-4 demonstrates the usefulness of somatosensory evoked response during a carotid endarterectomy in which a conscious patient experienced cerebral ischemia during carotid clamping [47]. Significant intraoperative SEP alterations have been correlated with postoperative decrements in neuropsychologic testing [48]. Amplitude reduction in SEPs postoperatively also correlated with worsening of neuropsychologic function in one series [49].

The SEP is easier to interpret than the EEG and, when compared bilaterally, the effects of anesthetics, changes in blood pressure, or equipment malfunction can be eliminated [47]. Inhalational anesthetics cause dose-related increases in the long-latency components and abolish them completely at high doses [50]. Short-latency components tend to be more resistant to moderate anesthetic concentrations.

Electroencephalogram

The EEG is a sensitive indicator of cerebral cortical function, but not of internal capsular or brainstem function. Although continuous multichannel EEG can be correlated with cerebral blood flow [51], the EEG does not show changes until cerebral metabolism is profoundly altered. No EEG changes are seen when cerebral blood flow remains above 30 ml/100 g/min, but definite changes occur below 18 ml/100 g/min [51]. Normally the frequency of the EEG, which is divided into alpha (8–13 Hz), beta (over 13 Hz), theta (4–7 Hz), and delta (0.5–3 Hz) bands, shifts from alpha, beta, and theta activity to delta activity with cerebral ischemia. Intraoperative depression of EEG amplitude is associated with postoperative cerebral damage. Its value in individual critical cases has been documented by Anderson et al. [52]. Wassman et al. [53] and Hansebout et al. [54] document its usefulness in detecting reversible signs of cerebral ischemia requiring shunt placement. In this respect, it is a more sensitive indicator than stump pressure.

However, the intraoperative EEG is also affected by depth of anesthesia, arterial Pco_2, muscle artifacts, and technical problems. The EEG increases in voltage during induction of general anesthesia and then decreases with deeper levels. There is also a shift of EEG activity from the occipital area to the frontal area, because occipital alpha activity is lost and frontal beta activity increases in amplitude. Decreasing arterial Pco_2 progressively slows the frequency of the EEG.

Computer-assisted EEG analysis and filter-processed EEG (cerebral function monitor) may detect changes when conventional EEG does not [55, 56] (figure 9-5 and figure 9-6). Even a lead system with one frontal ipsilateral lead and one contralateral mastoid lead analyzed by density spectral array demonstrated new intraoperative deficits in seven of 70 patients undergoing carotid endarterectomy [57].

Cerebral blood flow

Regional cerebral blood flow measurements reliably indicate cerebral ischemia. The measurement of regional cerebral blood flow using radioactive xenon washout curves remains a research technique not routinely applicable in most operating rooms. The critical level for cerebral blood flow appears to be 18–20 ml/100 g/min during inhalation anesthesia with normocarbia [58].

Intraoperative angiography and Doppler analysis

Although intraoperative angiography prolongs the operation and may increase the risk, it permits identification and correction of technical errors, which occur at frequencies of 5%–25% [59, 60]. However, only single-plane views are obtained, image quality is variable, and no information on physiologic flow is obtained. Since technical problems are infrequent when endarterectomies are performed frequently by skilled surgeons, intraoperative angiography is probably warranted only when endarterectomy is performed infrequently or during the learning phase of a surgeon [61].

A sterile pulsed Doppler spectral analysis detects technical problems accurately, obviating the need for routine and permitting selective intraoperative angiography [62]. The spectral assessment is improved over that obtained by

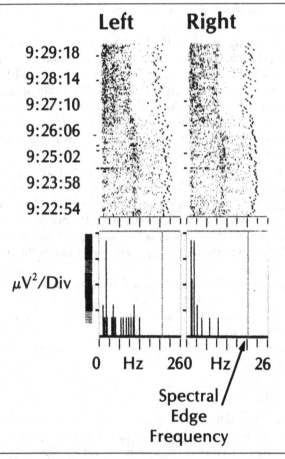

Figure 9-5. A density-modulated spectral array during left carotid endarterectomy. The spectral edge frequency is indicated. At 9:26, thiopental, 2 mg/kg, was given which decreased the high frequency activity of both cerebral hemispheres.

audible or analogue waveforms [62]. The Doppler can also monitor flow through an intraluminal shunt during endarterectomy.

PERIOPERATIVE MANAGEMENT

Only light premedication is necessary prior to general anesthesia for carotid endarterectomy, so neurologic status can be evaluated immediately prior to operation. Beta-adrenergic blockers and calcium entry-blocking drugs should be continued up to the time of surgery as withdrawal of beta-blockers results in a hyperdynamic state and often an increase in systemic vascular resistance [64]. Routine monitoring should include intraarterial pressure, electrocardiographic (ECG) leads II and V_5, and temperature to ensure cardiovascular stability during the procedure [63]. Hypertension is present in many patients

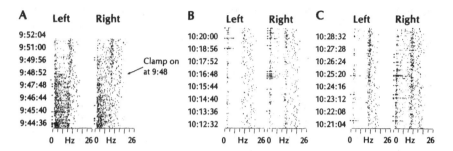

Figure 9-6. The density-modulated spectral array during left carotid endarterectomy.
A The left carotid artery is clamped at 9:48 with immediate decrease in frequency on the left side.
B Continued loss of left sided EEG activity with carotid occlusion.
C Partial return of EEG activity on the left with an increase in systemic arterial pressure and PCO_2. The patient had right hemiparesis post operatively.

with carotid disease. Both upper extremities should be evaluated to determine whether pressure differences exist. Radial arterial cannulation should be performed in the extremity with the higher pressure, assuming adequate collateral circulation is present.

In addition to the cerebral monitors discussed previously, transconjunctival oxygen tension and nasal plethysmography have been evaluated to monitor cerebral blood flow. Measurement of the conjunctival oxygen tension indicates manipulation, clamping, or obstruction of the ipsilateral carotid artery [65], but cannot be correlated with regional cerebral blood flow or EEG changes on carotid occlusion [66]. This discrepancy results from the vascular anatomy by which the conjunctival capillary bed is supplied not only by the ophthalmic branch of the internal carotid artery, but also by various branches of the external carotid artery [66]. The nasal plethysmograph also fails to correlate with direct cerebral blood flow measurements [67].

Significant coronary artery disease is also frequently present in patients with cerebrovascular disease. ECG lead V_5 monitors myocardial ischemia. Pulmonary artery catheters are indicated in patients with a history of severe myocardial dysfunction. Careful attention to the determinants of myocardial oxygen supply and demand as monitored by the ECG and arterial pressure is sufficient in most cases. However, the value of cardiac output and systemic vascular resistance measurements has been documented in patients with serious cardiac disease [68]. The transesophageal echocardiogram may eventually prove useful for assessing myocardial function during peripheral vascular procedures such as carotid endarterectomy.

CEREBRAL BLOOD FLOW

Cerebral blood flow is the difference between the systemic arterial pressure and the sum of intracranial and venous pressure. The normal mean cerebral blood flow is 46 ml/100 g/min, with flow to the grey matter at 80 ml/100 g/

min and to the white matter at 20 ml/100 g/min [69]. Major determinants of cerebral blood flow include carbon dioxide tension, oxygen tension, arterial blood pressure, local metabolic factors, and sympathetic nervous system activity [69, 70].

Cerebral blood flow is directly related to arterial P_{CO_2}. An arterial P_{CO_2} of less than 20 mmHg may diminish cerebral blood flow to a deleterious extent [71]. Over the range between 20 and 60 mmHg, cerebral blood flow is linearly related to P_{CO_2}, increasing 1 ml/100 g of brain for each 1 mmHg change in P_{CO_2} [72]. Autoregulation is partially preserved during hypocarbia, but is lost during hypercarbia [73].

Normocarbia limits both intracerebral steal and inverse steal phenomena. An elevated P_{CO_2} may dilate normal cerebral vessels, but not abnormal areas, leading to an intracerebral steal [73]. The converse is that a moderate decrease in P_{CO_2} may vasoconstrict relatively normal vessels, but not the abnormal ones. This event improves flow to ischemic areas—the "Robin Hood" phenomenon, or inverse steal.

Intense local production of lactic acid occurs in ischemic cerebral cells. The lactic acid stimulates local arteriolar vasodilatation—the luxury perfusion syndrome [75]. Sympathetic stimulation cerebral blood flow by 5%–10% while parasympathetic stimulation produces a slight vasodilator response [76].

Hyperoxia above a P_{O_2} of 50 torr has little effect on cerebral blood flow. Arterial P_{O_2} less than 50 mmHg increases cerebral blood flow and causes intracerebral lactic acidosis and cerebral vasodilatation [70]. The blood–brain barrier is resistant to hypoxia.

The carotid body, a group of oxygen-sensing cells near the carotid bifurcation, can also be damaged by carotid endarterectomy [77]. In systemic hypertension and left ventricular hypertrophy, the carotid bodies enlarge [78]. These structures, whose chief or glomus cells contain high concentrations of dopamine, are responsible for the reflex hyperpnea that occurs in response to acute hypoxia. They also reflexly respond to cause bradycardia and peripheral vasoconstriction, but this response is attenuated by general anesthesia [79]. Both the ventilatory and circulatory responses to hypoxia may be lost after bilateral carotid endarterectomy [77].

Cerebral blood flow is autoregulated over a wide range of arterial pressures between about 50 and 150 mmHg. Above about 180 mmHg, cerebral blood flow again becomes pressure dependent [70]. In patients with hypertension, the autoregulatory curve is shifted to the right so that both upper and lower limits of autoregulation are higher than in normotensives [76]. In hypertensive rats, hypotension with nitroprusside decreased cerebral blood flow more than in control or treated hypertensive rats [80]. Thus, control of hypertension may beneficially affect cerebral blood flow. Autoregulation is lost in areas of cerebral ischemia, making cerebral flow dependent upon perfusion pressure.

In addition to autoregulation, the brain is protected by collateral circulation through the circle of Willis, internal-to-external carotid anastomotic channels, and the occipital artery. During carotid occlusion, the adequacy of collateral flow depends upon the crossover flow through the circle of Willis, presence or absence of atherosclerotic disease in collateral vessels, and the systemic arterial pressure.

Hypothermia decreases the cerebral metabolic rate for oxygen (CMR_{O_2}) so that the EEG becomes isoelectric at 22°C. However, it is impractical to use hypothermia except with cardiopulmonary bypass because of the risk of ventricular fibrillation and the time necessary to induce and reverse sufficiently low temperatures.

Intravascular shunts

In an effort to provide nearly normal carotid flow, an intravascular shunt (Argyle or Javid) may be placed during carotid endarterectomy [73]. Anticoagulation with heparin, 1 mg/kg, is often used. The need for a shunt cannot be predicted from preoperative angiography [81] and its necessity is controversial. Surgeons may shunt routinely [82], selectively, or never [83]. Doppler flow studies, EEG, response to trial carotid occlusion [84], or the presence of preoperative contralateral carotid occlusive disease can be used to indicate the need for a shunt [53]. The flow through the shunt can be measured directly [85] or calculated indirectly, and is closely correlated with the difference between arterial pressure and stump pressure, but not with stump pressure itself [86]. The slope of the arterial pressure increase to carotid occlusion that correlates well with shunt blood flow may also indicate the necessity of a shunt [86]. Similar frequencies of neurologic deficit have been reported with or without shunts [87, 88].

The disadvantages of a shunt include difficulties in placement, including arterial dissection and dislodgement of atheromata, limitation of the surgical field, and the need for at least transient carotid occlusion for shunt placement [89, 90]. The majority of patients tolerate carotid clamping without shunting [91], so that only selective shunting should be performed. Criteria for shunting include prior cerebral infarction, reduced "stump pressure" (<25 torr), patients with reversible ischemic neurologic deficits or completed stroke, during general anesthesia, or when neurologic changes occur on occlusion in a patient under regional anesthesia. A shunt also permits unhurried surgery and acts as a stent during closure of the arteriotomy.

ANESTHETIC TECHNIQUES

Wells et al. [92] suggested general anesthesia with hypercarbia and induced hypertension as a preferred technique for carotid endarterectomy. They believed that this was protective because general anesthesia reduces oxygen consumption and easily increases arterial oxygen content, hypertension maintains blood flow through collateral channels, and hypercarbia increases cerebral blood flow [92]. Bailey and co-workers [93] recommended a similar technique with hypercarbia during halothane anesthesia, but this has been challenged because of the possibility of intracerebral steal and the increased incidence of cardiac arrhythmias [88]. At the present time, normocarbia, normotension, or slightly induced hypertension, mild systemic anticoagulation, normovolemia, and use of a volatile agent supplemented by nitrous oxide is the preferred technique.

INDUCTION AGENTS

There are two major ways to ameliorate hypoxic brain damage: (a) improve mitochondrial efficiency to optimize energy output during reduce oxygen supply, and (b) reduce overall metabolic activity [94]. Barbiturates decrease cerebral metabolic activity.

Thiopental decreases both CMR_{O_2} and cerebral blood flow, which may provide cerebral protection during ischemia [95–97]. McMeniman et al. [98] describe a series of patients in whom 4 mg/kg of thiopental was given prior to carotid clamping, followed by an infusion of 0.5 mg/kg/min during carotid occlusion, but there was no nonbarbiturate control group in their study.

Effects attributable to barbiturates include (a) protection during hypoxia [96, 99] (b) reduction of the extent of focal cerebral infarction in experimental animals [100] and in limited human trials [101], and (c) protection in global cerebral ischemia [101, 102]. However, because the protective effects of barbiturates in cerebral ischemia remain undocumented, it may be prudent to use them only when trial carotid occlusion results in EEG changes uncorrected by systemic pressure manipulation, shunt placement, or other therapeutic modalities. Loading doses of 2–75 mg/kg followed by infusion of 0.1–1.0 mg/kg/min have been used in these circumstances [103–106].

Of the other induction agents, ketamine also increases flow and cerebral metabolic rate for oxygen (CMR_{O_2}). Etomidate decreases CMR_{O_2} and is a cerebral vasoconstrictor [107]. Midazolam, a newly released water-soluble benzodiazepine, decreases CMR_{O_2} without systemic hemodynamic effects [108].

MAINTENANCE AGENTS

During the course of anesthesia, blood pressure should remain at control or higher levels, using small increments of phenylephrine or other vasoconstrictors if necessary [109]. Phenylephrine, metaraminol, dopamine, and norepinephrine do not change CMR_{O_2} if the blood–brain barrier remains intact [110]. However, the use of vasopressors in the subset of patients with heart disease increases the risk of perioperative myocardial infarction, even in patients operated using regional anesthesia [111]. Cerebral responsiveness to P_{CO_2} and pressure autoregulation are generally maintained except at very deep levels of anesthesia [112].

Halothane

Halothane increases cerebral blood flow. An isoelectric EEG occurs only at concentrations of halothane not tolerated by the cardiovascular system. However, unlike isoflurane, which favorably affects the cerebral energy state [113], halothane increases cerebral lactate–pyruvate ratio [114]. Halothane also attenuates the carotid sinus reflex changes in heart rate produced by changes in arterial pressure [115]. Cardiac sympathetic efferent activity decreases, while baroreceptor afferent activity is increased [115]. Postganglionic activity is more depressed than preganglionic, indicating a ganglionic blocking effect of halothane [115]. Pressor responses to bilateral carotid occlusion are depressed by halothane and completely suppressed at 1.3% end-tidal concentrations [116].

Enflurane

Enflurane also increases cerebral blood flow. The spike and dome complexes seen during deep enflurance anesthesia with hypocarbia and evidence of clinical seizure activity may relatively contraindicate its use during carotid endarterectomy. It is difficult to differentiate between seizures due to ischemia and an effect of enflurane.

Isoflurane

Isoflurane increases cerebral blood flow by decreasing cerebrovascular resistance [117]. However, in animals the associated induced decrease in $CMRo_2$ may be a protective mechanism, similar to that of barbiturates, during cerebral ischemia. [118]. Isoelectricity of the EEG occurs at 2 MAC isoflurane with $CMRo_2$ at about 50% of control [118].

Local anesthetics

The local anesthetic lidocaine can also be used to supplement nitrous oxide-narcotic anesthesia, providing about 30% of MAC [119]. It also decreases cerebral metabolic requirements and efflux of potassium from ischemic brain, and blocks sodium channels in high doses [120, 121].

Narcotics

Narcotics such as fentanyl, even in combination with droperidol, maintain cerebral blood flow and autoregulation [122]. Reactivity of the cerebral vasculature to carbon dioxide tension is also maintained.

Neuromuscular blocking drugs

Succinylcholine may be relatively contraindicated in patients with hemiplegia due to the possibility of hyperkalemia [123]. The use of nondepolarizing relaxants allows time to increase depth of anesthesia prior to endotracheal intubation, which decreases hypertension and tachycardia in patients with coronary disease.

HEMODYNAMIC CHANGES ASSOCIATED WITH CAROTID ENDARTERECTOMY

Control of arterial pressure (carotid sinus function)

Bilateral carotid occlusion in dogs increases systemic blood pressure and heart rate, but without any change in cardiac output or limb blood flow unless anemia is also induced [124]. Clamping of the carotid artery in dogs increases systemic vascular resistance and, a few seconds later, slightly decreases venous capacitance, an effect that is greater if vagal blockade is present [125].

Both hypotension and hypertension should be avoided in humans during carotid occlusion and reperfusion. Attainable goals should be no systolic blood pressures below 100 torr in normotensive patients or a greater than 40 torr decrease from the lowest preoperative systolic pressure in hypertensive individuals. The presence of intraoperative cerebral ischemia on EEG can frequently be reversed by induction of slight arterial hypertension [54]. Likewise, systolic pressures should remain less than 200 torr. In hypertensive patients, the baroreflex responses may be impaired [126]. Following carotid endarterectomy, about one-third of patients develop severe hypertension on emergence from anesthesia [127, 128], with a 79% incidence in those individuals with preoperative uncontrolled hypertension [129]. Hypertension secondary to carotid sinus dysfunction may be related to surgical dissection of the intercarotid (sinocarotid) nerves [130], preoperative uncontrolled hypertension, or a second carotid surgical procedure [130]. Changes in the mechanical properties of the arterial wall that increase its distensibility alter sinus nerve activity after endarterectomy [131]. An excellent response to carotid sinus nerve blockade has been reported [132]. However, the precise mechanism of postoperative hypertension is uncertain and the baroreceptor responses to surgery demonstrate considerable variability. In experimental rapid intracarotid infusions, damage to the blood–brain barrier accompanies acute elevations of carotid arterial pressure to 190 mmHg and increased cerebral blood flow [133].

NEUROLOGIC DEFICIT

Etiology

The incidence of neurologic deficit after surgery ranges between 1% and 7% [127, 134], regardless of anesthesia or surgical technique [128], including general anesthesia with hypercarbia but without a shunt, general anesthesia with a shunt, or regional anesthesia and trial occlusion (table 9-2). Neurologic deficits are increased in patients who are neurologically unstable preoperatively or have angiographically demonstrated risks, such as occlusion of the opposite internal carotid artery, stenosis of the internal carotid artery in the

Table 9-2. Complications of carotid endarterectomy

Cerebral neurologic deficits due to
  Emboli
  Thrombosis
  Hyperperfusion
Hypertension
Hypotension
Bradycardia
Seizures
Migraine variants
Local nerve damage (hypoglossal, laryngeal branches of vagus, greater auricular, and marginal
  mandibular branch of facial)

---

region of the siphon, extensive involvement of the operated vessel extending proximally and distally, and presence of soft thrombus extending from an ulcerated lesion [135]. Poorly controlled hypertension, postoperative hypertension [129, 136] (particularly greater than 200 torr [128]), surgical inexperience, prior stroke, extent of collaterals, duration of carotid clamping, and contralateral carotid disease were associated with neurologic deficits after operation [127]. A significant number of postoperative neurologic deficits are unrelated to ischemia secondary to inadequate cerebral collateral flow during carotid occlusion. They are instead due to emboli dislodged from atheromatous plaques during mobilization of vessels or insertion of shunts [87]. Development of a neurologic deficit after uneventful recovery from general anesthesia should be managed by immediate surgical reexploration [136]. Repeat angiography prior to reoperation is contraindicated. If a patent carotid is found, barbiturate therapy at 3–4 mg/kg/h for 36–48 h has been reported to be helpful [137].

Role of hyperperfusion

Another major cause of postoperative neurologic deficit is hyperperfusion resulting from increased cerebral blood flow. This commonly presents as transient seizures, migraine variants, and intracerebral hemorrhages [128]. It can be avoided by control of systemic arterial pressure, particularly in patients in whom cerebral autoregulation may be paralyzed (reversible ischemic neurologic deficits and recent CVA) [128]. In addition to cerebral neurologic impairment, there can be local nerve damage secondary to manipulation, pressure, or dissection during the endarterectomy. Among the nerves injured are: hypoglossal, the most commonly injured (9%); vagus (recurrent laryngeal branch, 6% incidence); vagus (superior laryngeal branch), glossopharyngeal, greater auricular nerve, and marginal mandibular branch of the facial nerve [138].

Role of anticoagulation

Reversal of anticoagulation with protamine does not increase the incidence of neurologic deficits compared with patients in whom heparin anticoagulation is permitted to terminate spontaneously [139]. Postoperative hemostasis is enhanced and no increase in the thrombogenicity of the endarterectomized vessel was noted. In fact, documentation of the state of coagulation periopera-tively using the Hemochron is warranted [140].

However, other recent studies suggest that immediate reversal of anticoagu-lation should not be performed upon reperfusion (carotid unclamping) [141]. Instead, the endarterectomized segment should be reperfused for at least 10 min, during which time a fibrin-free nonthrombogenic monolayer froms over the surface. With immediate reversal of heparin, or in the unanticoagulated state, there is fibrin and mural thrombus formation [141].

Management

It is not always clear whether postoperative hypertension is the result of or induces the complication of stroke. The presence of postoperative stroke also causes secondary hypertension, but this does not negate the need for blood pressure control. For these reasons, as well as the stress on a fresh arterial suture line, postoperative hypertension should be treated and controlled. A good response to vasodilators such as trimethaphan, nitroprusside, or hydrala-zine is often obtained.

Tarlov and co-workers [142] demonstrated hypotension and bradycardia in 41% of patients following carotid endarterectomy and attributed it to the undamped pressure wave reaching the carotid sinus after plaque removal. The sinus is then stimulated with an end result being the carotid sinus reflex. Atro-pine and phenylephrine or norepinephrine will counteract this syndrome. Catheter instillation of 2% lidocaine into the area of the carotid sinus post-operatively will also minimize postoperative hypotension [130, 143]. Other causes of hypotension such as underhydration, dysrhythmias, myocardial infarction, or blood loss should be evaluated and corrected before assuming that hypotension is the result of a baroreceptor response.

CONCLUSION

The choice of anesthesia for carotid endarterectomy is not clear-cut. Regional anesthesia is disadvantageous for carotid endarterectomy because of (1) the intraarterial injection of local anesthetic leading to convulsions; (2) neck mass-age to spread the anesthetic agents may cause cerebral emboli from plaques; (3) epinephrine may cause extrasystoles and palpitations; (4) injection of the hypo-glossal, phrenic, recurrent laryngeal, or facial nerves can be troublesome; (5) the airway is inaccessible if seizures develop; and (6) an uncooperative patient may make surgery difficult. However, a recent report notes no perioperative myocardial infarctions in a population of patients (25% with history of pre-vious myocardial infarction, 41% with documented coronary artery disease, and 75% with hypertension) who underwent carotid endarterectomy using superficial cervical plexus block anesthesia [144]. The need for routine carotid

Table 9-3. Advantages of general anesthesia for carotid endarterectomy

Better hemodynamic control
Improved oxygenation and airway control
More stable surgical field
Patient comfort and acceptance
Myocardial protection in patients with coronary artery disease
Increased cerebral protection (thiopental)
Rapidly changed to suit clinical conditions
0% failure rate

shunting is avoided by regional anesthesia as minute-to-minute neurologic monitoring of the conscious patient is possible. Observation of the conscious patient, whether intraoperatively or postoperatively, is more foolproof than any available cerebral monitor [38].

Another report [145] noted decreased overall hospital costs due to decreased intensive care unit and hospital stays, but also found higher systolic pressure intraoperatively when local anesthesia was used. Patients operated under local also required more pressor and antihypertensive than did those under general anesthesia [145]. This may relate to patient discomfort with stimulation of undesirable vagal and sympathetic responses. There are problems with these observations in that discharge from intensive care or need for it and hospital discharge may be subjective factors that are not born out by objective data in this study, where morbidity was the same in both local and general groups.

General anesthesia is preferable to regional since it reduces the risk of ischemia by allowing more complete control of blood pressure and systemic oxygenation (table 9-3). Both of these requirements are more important than the specific anesthetic drugs or agents used. In addition to providing a more stable operating field, which allows a more perfect endarterectomy, particularly exposure of the distal internal carotid artery, general anesthesia allows the administration to the patient of potentially cerebral-protective anesthetic agents. An incomplete or inadequate endarterectomy may be a greater factor in reduction of perioperative neurologic deficit. The general anesthetics capable of providing cerebral protection, of which thiopental is the prototype, do so by abolition of EEG activity. In addition, protection of the heart in these patients with associated coronary disease is present to a greater extent with general than with regional anesthesia, particularly in terms of avoiding hypoxia and hypercarbia and reducing myocardial oxygen demand. Greater control of arterial oxygenation is possible with general endotracheal anesthesia. Both heart and brain must be protected and the risks and benefits of specific techniques and drugs on each organ carefully weighed and modified to balance the risks. General anesthesia can be rapidly terminated at the end of the procedure, so that neurologic function can be assessed. It can also be rapidly changed in depth to suit clinical conditions, which is difficult or impossible with regional and local anesthesia. Although local anesthetics may have minimal organ system effects when given properly, the accidental intravascular (either arterial or venous) or intrathecal injection causes catastrophic hemodynamic and central nervous system events. In addition, general anesthesia has a 100% success rate, while 98% is probably the best that can be expected from local or regional anesthesia. Patient comfort is obviously greater with general than with regional anesthesia and may facilitate patient acceptance of the procedure.

Anesthesia per se probably plays a limited role, if any, in the outcome of carotid endarterectomy. The risk factors for perioperative stroke outlined by Imparato et al. [146] include technical problems (50%), intraoperative embolization (25%), intracerebral hemorrhage (16%), and other factors such as stroke in evolution and stroke from contralateral carotid, bradycardia, or myocardial infarction. A history of stroke and significant alterations of somatosensory evoked potentials intraoperatively, particularly in patients with bilateral carotid disease, have been associated with decrements in postoperative neuropsychologic performance [48]. Duration of ischemia (i.e., clamp time) was unassociated with poor postoperative neuropsychiatric testing [48]. Another series [147] noted that hypotension to a mean pressure less than 70 torr was associated with minor strokes and TIA in five of 184 patients, but that hypertension either intraoperatively or postoperatively was unassociated with such problems. Severe hypotension can cause postoperative vessel thrombosis.

Acute postoperative thrombosis is managed by rapid reexploration and reestablishment of cerebral flow if neurologic deficits are to be reversed. Extensive diagnostic procedures that delay surgery should not be performed [148].

Even with optimum perioperative management, the incidence of restenosis secondary to disease progression or myointimal hyperplasia is 12.5% [150]. The ultimate outcome from carotid surgery depends upon the presentation and pattern of disease in the individual, the rate of progression of atherosclerosis, and the presence of associated disease such as coronary artery disease [136].

REFERENCES

1. Carrea R, Molins M, Murphy G: Surgical treatment of spontaneous thrombosis of the internal carotid artery in the neck: carotid–carotideal anastomosis—report of case. Acta Neurol Lat Am 1:71–78, 1955.
2. Duncan GW, Pessin MS, Mohr JP, Adams RD: Transient cerebral ischemic attacks. Adv Intern Med 21:1–20, 1976.
3. Price TR, Gotshall RA, Poskanzer DC, Haerer AF, Swanson PD, Calanchini PR, Conneally PM, Dyken ML, Futty DE: Cooperative study of hospital frequency and character of transient ischemic attacks. JAMA 238:2512–2515, 1977.
4. Mentzer RM, Finkelmeier BA, Crosby IK, Wellons HA: Emergency carotid endarterectomy for fluctuating neurologic deficits. Surgery 89:60–66, 1981.
5. Roederer GO, Langlois YE, Lusiani L, Jager KA, Primozich J, Lawrence RJ, et al.: Natural history of carotid artery disease on the side contralateral to endarterectomy. J Vasc Surg 1:62–72, 1984.
6. Colgan MP, Kingston V, Shanik G: Asymptomatic carotid stenosis: is prophylactic endarterectomy justifiable? Br J Surg 72:313–314, 1985.

7. Quinones-Baldrich WJ, Moore WS: Asymptomatic carotid stenosis. Arch Neurol 42:378–382, 1985.
8. Clagett GP, Youkey JR, Brigham RA, Orecchia PM, Salander JM, Collins GJ, Rich NM: Asymptomatic cervical bruit and abnormal ocular pneumoplethysmography: a prospective study comparing two approaches to management. Surgery 96:823–830, 1984.
9. Dosick SM, Whalen RC, Gale SS, Brown OW: Carotid endarterectomy in the stroke patient: computerized axial tomography to determine timing. J Vasc Surg 2:214–219, 1985.
10. Fields WS, Lemak NA: Joint study of extracranial arterial occlusion. X. Internal carotid artery occlusion. JAMA 235:2734–2738, 1976.
11. Wylie EJ, Hein MF, Adams JE: Intracranial hemorrhage following surgical revascularization for treatment of acute strokes. J Neurosurg 21:212–215, 1964.
12. McCullough JL, Mentzer RM, Harman PK, Kaiser DL, Kron IL, Crosby IK: Carotid endarterectomy after a completed stroke: reduction in long-term neurologic deterioration. J Vasc Surg 2:7–14, 1985.
13. Brener BJ, Brief DK, Alpert J, Goldenkranz RJ, Parsonnet V, Feldman S, Gielchinsky I, Abel RM, Hochberg M, Hussain M: A four-year experience with preoperative noninvasive carotid evaluation of two thousand twenty-six patients undergoing cardiac surgery. J Vasc Surg 1:326–338, 1984.
14. Busuttil RW, Baker JD, Davidson RK, Machleder HI: Carotid artery stenosis: hemodynamic significance and clinical course. JAMA 245:1438–1441, 1981.
15. Gilroy J, Meyer JS: Auscultation of the neck in occlusive cerebrovascular disease. Circulation 25:300–310, 1962.
16. Chambers BR, Norris JW: Clinical significance of asymptomatic neck bruits. Neurology 35:742–745, 1985.
17. Balderman SC, Gutierrez IZ, Makula P, Bhayana JN, Gage AA: Noninvasive screening for asymptomatic carotid artery disease prior to cardiac operation. J Thorac Cardiovasc Surg 85:427–433, 1983.
18. Cebul RD, Ginsberg MD: Noninvasive neurovascular tests for carotid artery disease. Ann Intern Med 97:867–872, 1982.
19. Pence NA: Ophthalmodynamometry. J Am Optom Assoc 51:49–55, 1980.
20. Gee W, Mehigan JT, Wylie EJ: Measurement of collateral cerebral hemispheric blood pressure by ocular pneumoplethysmography. Am J Surg 130:121–127, 1975.
21. O'Hara PJ, Brewster DC, Darling RC, Hallett JW: Oculopneumoplethysmography. Arch Surg 115:1156–1158, 1980.
22. Kartchner MM, McRae LP, Crain V, Whitaker B: Oculoplethysmography: an adjunct to arteriography in the diagnosis of extracranial carotid occlusive disease. Am J Surg 132:728–732, 1976.
23. Kartchner NN, McRae LP, Morrison FD: Noninvasive detection and evaluation of carotid occlusive disease. Arch Surg 106:528–535, 1973.
24. Seeger JF, Carmody RF: Radiologic evaluation of the carotid arteries. CRC Crit Rev Diagn Imag 22:127–162, 1984.
25. Fuster B, Machado W, Vechi C: EEG and carotid cutaneous plethysmographic monitoring during carotid reconstructive surgery. Adv Neurol 30:379–392, 1981.
26. Uematsu S, Yang A, Preziosi TJ, Kouba R, Toung TJK: Measurement of carotid blood flow in man and its clinical application. Stroke 14:256–266, 1983.
27. Sundt TM, Sharbrough FW, Piepgras DG, Kearns TP, Messick JM, O'Fallon WM: Correlation of cerebral blood flow and electroencephalographic changes during carotid endarterectomy. Mayo Clin Proc 56:533–543, 1981.
28. Belkin M, Bucknam CA, Giuca JE, Horowitz LM: Combined oculoplethysmography and duplex scan. Arch Surg 120:809–811, 1985.
29. Jacobs NM, Grant EG, Schellinger D, Cohan SL, Byrd MC: The role of duplex carotid sonography, digital subtraction angiography, and arteriography in the evaluation of transient ischemic attack and the asymptomatic carotid bruit. Med Clin North Am 68:1423–1450, 1984.
30. Jacobs NM, Grant HG, Schellinger D, Byrd MC, Richarson JD, Cohan SL: Duplex carotid sonography: criteria for stenosis, accuracy, and pitfalls. Radiology 154:385–391, 1985.
31. Fitzgerald DE, O'Shaughnessy AM, Keaveny VT: Pulsed Doppler: determination of blood velocity and volume flow in normal and diseased common carotid arteries in man. Cardio-

vasc Res 16:220–224, 1982.

32. Archie JP, Feldman RW: Intraoperative assessment of carotid endarterectomy by electromagnetic blood flow measurements. Surg Gynecol Obstet 158:457–460, 1984.
33. Hacke W, Zeumer H, Ringelstein EB: EEG controlled occlusion of the internal carotid artery. Neuroradiology 22:19–22, 1981.
34. Ivey TD, Strandness DE, Williams DB, Langlois Y, Misbach GA, Kruse AP: Management of patients with carotid bruit undergoing cardiopulmonary bypass. J Thorac Cardiovasc Surg 87:183–189, 1984.
35. Zeumer H, Hundgen R, Ferbert A, Ringelstein EB: Local intrarterial fibrinolytic therapy in inaccessible internal carotid occlusion. Neuroradiology 26:315–317, 1984.
36. McKay RD, Sundt TM, Michenfelder JD, Gronert GA, Messick JM, Sharbrough FW, Piepgras DG: Internal carotid artery stump pressure and cerebral blood flow during carotid endarterectomy. Anesthesiology 45:390–399, 1976.
37. Bergan JJ: Extracranial vascular surgery. Surg Annu 13:53–74, 1981.
38. Kwaan JH, Peterson GJ, Connolly JE: Stump pressure: an unreliable guide for shunting during carotid endarterectomy. Arch Surg 115:1083–1086, 1980.
39. Ricotta JJ, Charlton MH, Deweese JA: Determining criteria for shunt placement during carotid endarterectomy. Ann Surg 198:642–645, 1983.
40. Ehrenfeld WK, Larson CP, Fourcade HE, Wylie EJ: Hypocarbic anesthesia during carotid endarterectomy. Surg Forum 21:420–423, 1970.
41. Fourcade HF, Larson CP, Ehrenfeld WK, Hickey RF Newton TH: The effects of carbon dioxide and systemic hypertension on cerebral perfusion pressure during carotid endarterectomy. Anesthesiology 33:383–390, 1970.
42. Sublett JW, Seidenberg AB, Hobson RW: Internal carotid artery stump pressure during regional anesthesia. Anesthesiology 41:505–508, 1974.
43. Larson CP, Ehrenfeld WK, Wade JG, Wylie EJ: Jugular venous oxygen saturation as an index of adequacy of cerebral oxygenation. Surgery 62:31–39, 1967.
44. Grundy BL: Intraoperative monitoring of sensory-evoked potentials. Anesthesiology 58: 72–87, 1983.
45. Branston NM, Symon L, Crockard HA: Relationship between cortical evoked potential and local cortical blood flow following acute middle cerebral artery occlusion in the baboon. Exp Neurol 45:195–208, 1974.
46. Markand ON, Dilley RS, Warren C: Monitoring of somatosensory evoked responses during carotid endarterectomy. Arch Neurol 41:375–378, 1984.
47. Moorthy SS, Markand ON, Dilley RS, McCammon RL, Warren CH: Somatosensory evoked responses during carotid endarterectomy. Anesth Analg 61:879–883, 1982.
48. Cushman L, Brinkman SD, Ganji S, Jacobs LA: Neuropsychological impairment after carotid endarterectomy correlates with intraoperative ischemia. Cortex 20:403–412, 1984.
49. Brinkman SD, Braun P, Ganji S, Morrell RM, Jacobs LA: Neuropsychological performance one week after carotid endarterectomy reflects intra-operative ischemia. Stroke 15:497–503, 1984.
50. Uhl RR, Squires KC, Bruce DL, Starr A: Effect of halothane anesthesia on the human cortical evoked response. Anesthesiology 53:273–276, 1980.
51. Sharbrough FW, Messick JM, Sundt TM: Correlation of continuous electroencephalograms with cerebral blood flow measurements during carotid endarterectomy. Stroke 4:674–683, 1973.
52. Anderson EM, Carney AL, Page L: Carotid and vertebral artery surgery, EEG monitoring, and the operating room. Adv Neurol 30:361–377, 1981.
53. Wassman H, Fischdick G, Jain KK: Cerebral protection during carotid endarterectomy: EEG monitoring as a guide to the use of intraluminal shunts. Acta Neurochir (Wien) 71:99–108, 1984.
54. Hansebout RR, Blomquist G, Gloor P, Thompson C, Trop D: Use of hypertension and electroencephalographic monitoring during carotid endarterectomy. Can J Surg 24:304–307, 1981.
55. Cucchiara RF, Sharbrough FW, Messick JM, Tinker JH: An electroencephalographic filter processor as an indicator of cerebral ischemia during carotid endarterectomy. Anesthesiology 51:77–79, 1979.
56. Grundy BL, Sanderson AC, Webster MW, Richey ET, Procopio P, Karanjia PN: Hemi-

paresis following carotid endarterectomy: comparison of monitoring methods. Anesthesiology 55:462–466, 1981.

57. Rampil IJ, Holzer JA, Quest DO, Rosenbaum SH, Correll JW: Prognostic value of computerized EEG analysis during carotid endarterectomy. Anesth Analg 62:186–192, 1983.

58. Boysen G, Engell HC, Pistolese GR, Fiorani P, Agnoli A, Lassen NA: On the critical lower level of cerebral blood flow in man with particular reference to carotid surgry. Circulation 49:1023–1025, 1974.

59. Blaisdell FW, Lin R, Hall AD: Technical result of carotid endarterectomy: an arteriographic assessment. Am J Surg 114:239–246, 1967.

60. Rosental JJ, Gaspar MR, Mavius HJ: Intraoperative arteriography in carotid thromboendarterectomy. Arch Surg 106:806–808, 1973.

61. Jernigan WR, Fulton RL, Hamman JL, Miller FB, Mani SS: The efficacy of routine completion operative angiography in reducing the incidence of perioperative stroke associated with carotid endarterectomy. Surgery 96:831–837, 1985.

62. Zierler RE, Bandyk DF, Thiele BL: Intraoperative assessment of carotid endarterectomy. J Vasc Surg 1:73–83, 1984.

63. Jenkins LC, Chung WB: Clinical appraisal of adequacy of brain circulation during anesthesia with particular reference to carotid thromboendarterectomy. Can Anaesth Soc J 16:461–476, 1969.

64. Pontén J, Biber B, Henriksson B-Å, Hjalmarson Å, Jonsteg C, Lundberg B: Beta receptor blockade and neurolept anaesthesia: withdrawal vs continuation of long-term therapy in gall bladder and carotid artery surgery. Acta Anaesth Scand 26:576–588, 1982.

65. Shoemaker WC, Lawner PM: Method for continuous conjunctival oxygen monitoring during carotid artery surgery. Crit Care Med 11:946–947, 1983.

66. Gibson BE, McMichan JC, Cucchiara RF: Lack of correlation between transconjunctival O_2 and cerebral blood flow during carotid artery occlusion. Anesthesiology 64:277–279, 1986.

67. Cucchiara RF, Messick JM: The failure of nasal plethysmography to estimate cerebral blood flow during carotid occlusion. Anesthesiology 55:585–586, 1981.

68. Pritz MB, Kindt GW: Perioperative management of high risk patients with cardiopulmonary disease undergoing carotid endarterectomy or extracranial–intracranial bypass. Neurosurgery 10:442–427, 1982.

69. Smith AL, Wollman H: Cerebral blood flow and metabolism. Anesthesiology 36:378–400, 1972.

70. Lassen NA: Control of cerebral circulation in health and disease. Circ Res 34:749–760, 1974.

71. Michenfelder JD, Sundt TM: The effect of $Paco_2$ on the metabolism of ischemic brain in squirrel monkeys. Anesthesiology 38:445–453, 1973.

72. Kety SS, Schmidt CF: The effects of altered tensions of carbon dioxide and oxygen on cerebral blood flow and cerebral oxygen consumption of normal young men. J Clin Invest 27:484–492, 1948.

73. Boysen G: Cerebral hemodynamics in carotid surgery. Acta Neurol Scand [Suppl 52] 49: 15–58, 1973.

74. Symon L: Regional cerebrovascular responses to acute ischaemia in normocapnia and hypercapnia. J Neurol Neurosurg Psychiatry 33:756–762, 1970.

75. Lassen NA: The luxury perfusion syndrome and its possible relation to acute metabolic acidosis localized within the brain. Lancet 2:1113–1115, 1966.

76. Lassen NA, Christensen MS: Physiology of cerebral blood flow. Br J Anaesth 48:719–734, 1976.

77. Lee JK, Hanowell S, Kim YD, Macnamara TE: Morphine-induced respiratory depression following bilateral carotid endarterectomy. Anesth Analg 61:64–65, 1981.

78. Gronblad M: Function and structure of the carotid body. Med Biol 61:229–248, 1983.

79. Zimpfer M, Sit SP, Vatner SF: Effects of anesthesia on the canine carotid chemoreceptor reflex. Circ Res 48:400–406, 1981.

80. Hoffman WE, Miletich DJ, Albrecht RF: Cerebrovascular response to hypotension in hypertensive rats: effects of antihypertensive therapy. Anesthesiology 58:326–332, 1983.

81. Ward R, Flynn T, Kelly JT, Reilly E, Handel S: Electroencephalogram monitoring during carotid endarterectomy. J Cardiovasc Surg 22:127–133, 1981.

82. Schiro J, Mertz GH, Cannon JA, Cintora I: Routine use of a shunt for carotid endarterec-

tomy. Am J Surg 142:735–738, 1981.

83. Whitney DG, Kahn EM, Estes JW, Jones CE: Carotid artery surgery without a temporary indwelling shunt. Arch Surg 115:1393–1399, 1980.
84. Steed DL, Peitzman AB, Grundy BL, Webster MW: Causes of stroke in carotid endarterectomy. Surgery 92:634–641, 1982.
85. Lindsey RL: A simple solution for determining shunt flow during carotid endarterectomy. Anesthesiology 61:215–216, 1984.
86. Fan F-C, Chen RYZ, Chien S, Correll JW: Bypass blood flow during carotid endarterectomy. Anesthesiology 55:305–310, 1981.
87. Rosenthal D, Zeichner WD, Lamis PA, Stanton PE: Neurologic deficit after carotid endarterectomy: pathogenesis and management. Surgery 94:776–780, 1983.
88. Baker WH, Rodman RA, Barnes RW, Hoyt JL: An evaluation of hypocarbia and hypercarbia during carotid endarterectomy. Stroke 7:451–454, 1976.
89. Akl BF, Blakeley WR, Lewis CE, Edward WS: Carotid endarterectomy: is a shunt necessary? Am J Surg 130:760–765, 1975.
90. Calhoun TR, Kitten CM: Proximal shunt dissection: a potential problem in carotid endarterectomy. Tex Heart Inst J 12:359–361, 1985.
91. Chiappa KH, Burke SR, Young RR: Results of electroencephalographic monitoring during 367 carotid endarterectomies. Stroke 10:381–388, 1979.
92. Wells BA, Keats AS, Cooley DA: Increased tolerance to cerebral ischemia produced by general anesthesia during temporary carotid occlusion. Surgery 54:216–223, 1963.
93. Bailey LL, Driggs BD, Smith LI: Systemic hemodynamic changes during hypercarbic halothane anesthesia for carotid endarterectomy. Anesth Analg 50:217–221, 1971.
94. Graham DI: The pathology of brain ischaemia and possibilities for therapeutic intervention. Br J Anaesth 57:3–17, 1985.
95. Michenfelder JD, Milde JH: Influence of anesthetics on metabolic, functional and pathological responses to regional cerebral ischemia. Stroke 6:405–410, 1975.
96. Michenfelder JD, Milde JH, Sundt TM: Cerebral protection by barbiturate anesthesia. Arch Neurol 33:345–350, 1976.
97. Smith AL, Hoff JT, Nielsen SL, Larson CP: Barbiturate protection in acute focal cerebral ischemia. Stroke 5:1–7, 1974.
98. McMeniman WJ, Fletcher JP, Little JM: Experience with barbiturate therapy for cerebral protection during carotid endarterectomy. Ann R Coll Surg Engl 66:361–364, 1984.
99. Steen PA, Michenfelder JD: Barbiturate protection in tolerant and non-tolerant hypoxic mice: comparison with hypothermic protection. Anesthesiology 50:404–408, 1979.
100. Michenfelder JD, Milde JH, Sundt JM Jr: Cerebral protection by barbiturate anesthesia: use after middle cerebral artery occlusion in Java monkeys. Arch Neurol 33:345–350, 1976.
101. Rockoff MA, Marshall LF, Shapiro HM: High dose barbiturate therapy in humans: a clinical review of 60 patients. Ann Neurol 6:194–199, 1979.
102. Bleyaert AL, Nemoto EM, Safar P, Stezoski SW, Mickell JJ, Moossy J, Rao GR: Thiopental amelioration of brain damage after global ischemia in monkeys. Anesthesiology 49:390–398, 1978.
103. Becker DP, Miller JD, Ward JD, Greenberg RP, Young HF, Sakalas R: The outcome from severe head injury with early diagnosis and intensive head management. J Neurosurg 47:491–502, 1977.
104. Moffat JA, McDougall MJ, Brunet B, Saunders F, Shelly ES, Cervenko FW, Milne B: Thiopental bolus during carotid endarterectomy: rational drug therapy. Can Anaesth Soc J 30:615–622, 1983.
105. Spetzler RF, Selman WR, Roski RA, Bonstelle C: Cerebral revascularization during barbiturate coma in primates and humans. Surg Neurol 17:111–115, 1982.
106. Todd MM, Chadwick HS, Shapiro HM, Dunlop BJ, Marshall LF, Dueck R: The neurologic effects of thiopental therapy following experimental cardiac arrest in cats. Anesthesiology 57:76–86, 1982.
107. Wauquier A: Profile of etomidate: a hypnotic, anticonvulsant and brain protective compound. Anaesthesia [Suppl] 38:26–33, 1983.
108. Nugent M, Artru AA, Michenfelder JD: Cerebral metabolic, vascular, and protective effects of midazolam maleate. Anesthesiology 56:172–176, 1982.
109. Fitch W: Anaesthesia for carotid artery surgery. Br J Anaesth 48:791–796, 1976.

110. Gevarghese KP: Basic considerations. Int Anesthesiol Clin 15(3):1–56, 1977.
111. Riles TS, Kopelman I, Imparato AM: Myocardial infarction following carotid endarterectomy: a review of 683 operations. Surgery 85:249–252, 1979.
112. Boysen G, Ladegaard-Pedersen HJ, Henriksen H, Olesen J, Paulson OB, Engell HC: The effects of $Paco_2$ on regional cerebral blood flow and internal carotid arterial pressure during carotid clamping. Anesthesiology 35:286–300, 1971.
113. Newberg LA, Michenfelder JD: Cerebral protection by isoflurane during hypoxemia or ischemia. Anesthesiology 59:29–35, 1983.
114. Michenfelder JD, Theye RA: In vivo toxic effects of Halothane on canine cerebral metabolic pathways. Am J Physiol 229:1050–1055, 1975.
115. Seagard JL, Hopp FA, Donegan JH, Kalbfleisch JH, Kampine JP: Halothane and the carotid sinus reflex. Anesthesiology 57:191–202, 1982.
116. Bagshaw RJ, Cox RH: Effects of incremental halothane levels on the reflex responses to carotid hypotension in the dog. Acta Anaesth Scand 25:180–184, 1981.
117. Cucchiara RF, Theye RA, Michenfelder JD: The effects of isoflurane on canine cerebral metabolism and blood flow. Anesthesiology 40:571–574, 1974.
118. Newberg LA, Milde JH, Michenfelder JD: The cerebral metabolic effects of isoflurane at and above concentrations that suppress cortical electrical activity. Anesthesiology 59:23–28, 1983.
119. Himes RS, DiFazio CA, Burney RG: Effect of lidocaine on the anesthetic requirements for nitrous oxide and halothane. Anesthesiology 47:437–440, 1977.
120. Astrup J: Energy-requiring cell functions in the ischemic brain. J Neurosurg 56:482–497, 1982.
121. Astrup J, Moller Sorensen P, Rahbeck Sorenson H: Inhibition of cerebral oxygen and glucose consumption in the dog by hypothermia, pentobarbital and lidocaine. Anesthesiology 55:263, 1981.
122. Klintmalm G, Astrom H, Bergenwald L, Cronestrand R, von Euler C, Juhlin-Dannfelt AJ: Intraoperative variation in carotid artery blood flow and cardiac output: the effects of changes in blood volume and carbon dioxide during surgery under neurolept anesthesia. Acta Chir Scand 148:121–125, 1982.
123. Cooperman LH, Strobel GE, Kennell EM: Massive hyperkalemia after administration of succinylcholine. Anesthesiology 32:161–164, 1970.
124. Cain SM, Chapler CK: Cardiovascular and metabolic responses to carotid clamping in anemic dogs. Adv Exp Med Biol 169:381–387, 1984.
125. Bennett TD, Wyss CR, Scher AM: Changes in vascular capacity in awake dogs in response to carotid sinus occlusion and administration of catecholamines. Circ Res 55:440–453, 1984.
126. Lindblad LE, Bevegård S, Castenfors J, Tranesjö J: Circulatory effects of carotid sinus stimulation and changes in blood volume distribution in hypertensive man. Acta Physiol Scand 111:299–306, 1981.
127. Asiddao CB, Donegan JH, Whitesell RC, Kalbfleisch JH: Factors associated with perioperative complications during carotid endarterectomy. Anesth Analg 61:631–637, 1982.
128. Sabawala PB, Strong MJ, Keats AS: Surgery of the aorta and its branches. Anesthesiology 3:229–259, 1970.
129. Towne JB, Bernhard VM: The relationship of postoperative hypertension to complications following carotid endarterectomy. Surgery 88:575–580.
130. Cafferata HT, Merchant RF, DePalma RG: Avoidance of postcarotid endarterectomy hypertension. Ann Surg 196:465–472, 1982.
131. Angell-James JE, Lumley JSP: The effects of carotid endarterectomy on the mechanical properties of the carotid sinus and carotid sinus nerve activity in atherosclerotic patients. Br J Surg 61:805–810, 1974.
132. Tyden G, Somnegard H, Thulin L: Rational treatment of hypotension after carotid endarterectomy by carotid sinus nerve blockade. Acta Chir Scand [Suppl] 500:61–64, 1980.
133. Hardebo JE, Nilsson B: Opening of the blood brain barrier by acute elevation of intracarotid pressure. Acta Physiol Scand 111:43–49, 1981.
134. Thompson JE: Carotid endarterectomy, 1982: the state of the art. Br J Surg 70:371–376, 1983.
135. Sundt TM: Ischemic tolerance of neural tissue and the need for monitoring and selective shunting during carotid endarterectomy. Stroke 14:93–98, 1983.

136. Lehv MS, Salzman EW, Silen W: Hypertension complicating carotid endarterectomy. Stroke 1:307–313, 1970.
137. Markowitz IP, Adinolfi MF, Kerstein MD: Barbiturate therapy in the postoperative endarterectomy patient with a neurologic deficit. Am J Surg 148:221–223, 1984.
138. Lusby RJ, Wylie EJ: Complications of carotid endarterectomy. Surg Clin North Am 63: 1293–1302, 1983.
139. Chandler WF, Ercius MS, Ford JW, LaBond V, Burkel WE: The effect of heparin reversal after carotid endarterectomy in the dog. J Neurosurg 56:97–102, 1982.
140. Rosenwasser RH, Garrido E, Freed MH, Shupak RC: Monitoring of activated clotting time during carotid endarterectomy: a preliminary report. Neurosurgery 9:521–523, 1981.
141. Ercius MS, Chandler WF, Ford JW, Burkel WE: Early versus delayed heparin reversal after carotid endarterectomy in the dog. J Neurosurg 58:708–713, 1983.
142. Tarlov E, Schmidek H, Scott RM, Wepsic JG, Ojemann RG: Reflex hypotension following carotid endarterectomy: mechanism and management. J Neurosurg 39:323–327, 1973.
143. Pine R, Avellone JC, Hoffman M, Plecha R, Swayngim M, Urban J: Control of postcarotid endarterectomy hypotension with baroreceptor blockade. Am J Surg 147:763–765, 1984.
144. Prough DS, Scuderi PE, Stullken E, Davis CH: Myocardial infarction following regional anesthesia for carotid endarterectomy. Can Anaesth Soc J 31:192–196, 1984.
145. Gabelman CG, Gann, DS, Ashworth CJ, Carney WI: One hundred consecutive carotid reconstructions: local versus general anesthesia. Am J Surg 145:447–482, 1983.
146. Imparato AM, Ramirez A, Riles T, Mintzer R: Cerebral protection in carotid surgery. Arch Surg 117:1073–1078, 1982.
147. Owens ML, Wilson SE: Prevention of neurologic complications. Arch Surg 117:551–555, 1982.
148. Novick WM, Millili JJ, Nemir P: Management of acute postoperative thrombosis following carotid endarterectomy. Arch Surg 120:922–925, 1985.

10. REGIONAL ANESTHESIA IS PREFERABLE FOR PATIENTS UNDERGOING CAROTID ENDARTERECTOMY

PIERRE CASTHELY AND JOHN DLUZNESKI

Strokes are the third leading cause of death in North America [1]. They usually result from arterial occlusive disease involving the extracranial or intracranial vessels, or both, in 80% of the cases; 35%–40% of the patients with cerebrovascular insufficiency have significant intracranial vascular disease [2]. The site of occlusion may be extracranial or intracranial. Cerebral ischemia can be produced either by embolic infarction or by reducing cerebral perfusion. The source of most of the embolic material producing transient ischemic attacks (TIAs) and stroke appears to be platelet and fibrin–platelet casts, formed at the site of an atherosclerotic plaque, which then migrate into the intracranical vessels. This is the reasoning behind using aspirin, which inhibits platelet aggregation, in that group of patients.

Medical management is aimed at establishing the presence of cerebrovascular occlusive disease and treating it before a stroke occurs. It consists mainly of treatment of conditions [2] associated with high risk of strokes such as obesity, arteriosclerosis, and arterial hypertension. The place of vasodilators, salicylates, and anticoagulants is still uncertain. There is no proof that stellate ganglion blocks are of benefit in these cases. Of the patients with stroke, 55%–75% are hypertensive. Isolated systolic hypertension increases the risk of stroke 2–6 times over that in normotensive age-matched individuals [3]. Antihypertensive therapy can prevent or delay the initial or recurrent stroke [4], as well as reduce the incidence of many other complications of hypertension. Other risk factors for stroke include diabetes, smoking, peripheral vascular disease, hyperlipemia, and impaired cardiac function [2]; 30%–40% of patients will have a history of one or more TIAs as a warning sign [5]. The fact that most intracranial vascular lesions are at the carotid bifurcation has made carotid endarterectomy a common surgical procedure.

Indications for this procedure include (a) TIAs (including amaurosis fugax), (b) mild stable stroke with good neurologic recovery and (c) selected cases of asymptomatic carotid bruit. Most surgeons would operate on a patient who had a significant carotid lesion and an associated TIA or a completed stroke with good recovery. Acute profound stroke, stroke in progress, and severe intracranial disease are contraindications for surgery because of the high incidence of postoperative hemorrhagic infarctions. The role of reconstructive surgery in management of patients with asymptomatic carotid stenosis is not clear. Two studies showed no incidence of perioperative TIA or stroke in patients with asymptomatic carotid bruits who underwent coronary artery bypass and major peripheral vascular procedures [6, 7].

ANATOMY

The brain has a rich blood supply, the most important being the circle of Willis [8]. When a carotid artery is 50% occluded, adequate cerebral perfusion can be easily maintained through the contralateral carotid or the vertebral arteries. Other important arterial collaterals are available through the proximal internal carotid via the opthalmic or occipital artery to the distal internal carotid artery.

DIAGNOSIS

Cerebral angiography preferably performed via the femoral route, with visualization of both the carotid and the vertebral systems, remains the most reliable diagnostic test for patients with cerebrovascular insufficiency. Angiographically defined risk factors include (a) occlusion of the opposite internal carotid artery (ICA), (b) stenosis of the ICA in the region of the siphon, (c) extensive involvement of the vessel to be operated on, with extension of the plaque distally in the ICA, (d) bifurcation of the carotid artery at C_2 in conjunction with a short, thick neck, and (e) evidence of a soft thrombus extending from an ulcerative lesion [7]. A number of relatively new nonivasive tests have been developed for evaluating the cerebral circulation. These include the Doppler examination, opthalmodynamometery, oculoplethysmography, and photoplethysmography. Indications for noninvasive carotid evaluation include (a) patients with typical TIAs but relative contraindications to arteriography, (b) patients with a previous stroke with good recovery, (c) patients with asymptomatic carotid bruits, and (d) patients with central retinal artery occlusion.

CEREBRAL DAMAGE FROM CAROTID ENDARTERECTOMY

Cerebral damage from carotid endarterectomy occurs because of dislodgement of emboli from stenosis site and reduction in regional perfusion because of surgical emboli, clamping, or occlusion.

It is now recognized that dislodged emboli probably play a major role in the pathogenesis of TIA and focal cerebral damage associated with carotid artery stenosis and carotid artery surgery [9]. This may result from repeated palpation of the neck vessels preoperatively or during surgical dissection of the carotid with palpation [10].

REDUCTION OF PERFUSION

Hypotension of even minor magnitude, anytime, in the presence of carotid stenosis can jeopardize blood flow to the affected area. It does so by altering the perfusion efficiency of the circle of Willis and the collateral circulation [11].

The effect of temporary carotid clamping on cerebral blood has been studied by many investigators using regional blood flow (rCBF) measurements [11–13]. They have demonstrated that temporary clamping of the carotid artery reduced rCBF by 4% in most patients. Autoregulation to reduction in perfusion pressure has been reported to be instantaneous. It was noted that hemispheric flow fell immediately on clamping, followed by a further reduction during the next 10–20 s, and thereafter remaining constant for the next 20 min [11, 14].

This reduction in cerebral blood flow can be compensated for by one of two approaches: use of a shunt or evaluation of cerebral hemodynamics during and after endarterectomy.

SHUNT

Carotid artery bypass shunts are used by many surgeons to maintain blood flow to the ICA during cross-clamping. In about two-thirds of patients, the shunt is not necessary. Disadvantages of a shunt include extension of operative time for shunt placement, larger surgical incision, partial obstruction of the surgical field, and its placement and removal uses time during which carotid flow must be occluded. Complications resulting from shunt placement that can increase morbidity include thromboembolism, air embolism, intimal dissection, and shunt clotting. Because of these complications, surgeons are very selective as to when to use a shunt.

Regional anesthesia offers the perfect way to monitor adequacy of cerebral blood flow and cerebral deterioration during the most critical period of carotid artery surgery, which is during the cross-clamping of the carotid artery.

PREOPERATIVE EVALUATION AND PREPARATION

Atherosclerosis is a generalized disease. Most patients who have carotid artery stenosis will have some degree of coronary artery disease. Sundt and associates [15] examined the factors related to outcome following carotid endarterectomy. They concluded that the major medical risk factors were angina pectoris, myocardial infarction of less than 6 months' duration, congestive heart failure, blood pressure greater than 180/100 mmHg, chronic obstructive pulmonary disease, age over 70 years, and marked obesity.

Several points deserve special attention:

1. A thorough cardiovascular examination must be performed with an electro-cardiogram and routine laboratory studies.
2. As blood pressure is often labile, it should be frequently measured and the full range of pressures determined.
3. Pressure should be measured in both arms and with the patients in various positions. Hypertension presents a special risk.
4. Peripheral pulses should be located prior to placement of arterial catheters (Allen's test or Ramanathan test).
5. Do not palpate carotid arteries, as cerebral embolism may occur.
6. A good neurologic examination must be performed and the results of any noninvasive tests, including cerebral angiography, must be reviewed. A patient with narrowed vertebral arteries in addition to carotid disease may be particularly intolerant to changes in head position. Facial pulses should also be evaluated [16].
7. All preoperative medications should be continued up to the day of surgery. Abrupt discontinuation of clonidine may cause rebound hypertension that can be difficult to control.
8. Since sensorium monitoring is important while the carotid is clamped, heavy preoperative and intraoperative medication is not recommended during regional anesthesia.

The adequacy of cerebral perfusion can be measured by jugular venous oxygen saturation [17], electroencephalogram [18], rCBF measurements [18], stump pressure [19], noninvasive carotid studies (oculoplethysmography and photoplethysmography) [20], and evoked potentials [20].

ANESTHETIC CONSIDERATIONS

The major concern during carotid endarterectomy is the prevention of cerebral damage that may result from embolic phenomena or from a reduction in cerebral perfusion. Since dislodgement of emboli is most frequently due to surgical dissection and shunt insertion, the major goal of optimal anesthestic management is the avoidance of a reduction in perfusion pressure. The anesthesiologist must know about factors regulating cerebral blood flow, autoregulation, chemical control of cerebral blood flow, and neurogenic control of cerebral blood flow. Since many of those patients have myocardial ischemia, the relationship between myocardial oxygen supply and demand should be optimized.

The choice of anesthesia for carotid endarterectomy is not a clear one. One has to consider the risk of a postoperative myocardial infarction, bleeding, or cerebral vascular accident. In addition, adequacy of cerebral perfusion and oxygenation should be assessed intraoperatively.

JUGULAR VENOUS OXYGEN SATURATION

Jugular venous oxygen saturation (SV_{O_2}) has been reported as a useful indicator of cerebral perfusion during carotid endarterectomy. Lyons et al. [22] suggested that a jugular venous S_{O_2} of 50% was acceptable as a criteria for the adequacy of cerebral perfusion. However, the validity of jugular venous content of oxygen or brain metabolites, such as lactate and pyruvate, is not questioned, since mixing of blood from both cerebral hemispheres is known to occur.

ELECTROENCEPHALOGRAM RECORDING

Routine electroencephalogram (EEG) recordings could be normal in patients with a history if TIA unless taken during or immediately after an attack. When preoperative focal ischemia is present, it is likely to be evident in the EEG. Preoperative EEG monitoring has been employed as a test of collateral function using test occlusion by digital compression of the involved carotid artery and simultaneous EEG recordings [10, 24]. A critical reduction of cerebral perfusion brought about by occlusion of the involved side leads to EEG changes [25]. There was a close relationship between EEG changes and clinical signs of ischemia in awake patients under local anesthesia. Digital carotid compression is not without complications of its own such as bradycardia, embolization, and sometimes thrombosis of the carotid artery [26, 27] (M. Atik, personal communication, 1973).

Intraoperative EEG changes have been correlated with rCBF measurements and ICA pressure during carotid clamping [28]. In all the patients who developed EEG changes during carotid occlusion, the internal carotid stump pressure was below 50 mmHg. Patients who had low rCBF preoperatively showed no EEG changes on clamping, but showed higher ICA stump pressures. EEG changes occurred within 20–40 s after occlusion in almost all of the patients.

Recognizing the gross flattening of the EEG that results from severe reduction in cerebral perfusion is an easy task. However, minor EEG changes are difficult to interpret in view of the superimposed effects of oxygenation upon EEG. Multiple-lead EEG is still a research tool that is not yet a common routine during carotid endarterectomy.

REGIONAL CEREBRAL BLOOD FLOW

Tolerance of the human brain to ischemia has not been determined. The minimum rCBF required during carotid clamping is now known. When compared to all the other techniques employed to study the hemodynamic changes related to carotid artery occlusion and to evaluate the reliability of the various methods in detecting cerebral vascular insufficiency, rCBF measurements are the most sophisticated. The most common method of study of rCBF is the technique of ^{133}Xe intraarterial injection described by Lassen [12, 13]. Washout of the tracer injected into the internal carotid artery above the level of the lesion following surgical exposure can be recorded from the brain either by a simple scintillation detector, or by a multichannel system of scintillation detectors collimated individually, which allows each detector to see only a predetermined region of the hemisphere. Measurements of rCBF, to be meaningful, should be made preoperatively following surgical exposure of the carotid artery during a test occlusion of 2 minutes of the common and external carotid and then following endarterectomy. Measurements could also be obtained with a shunt in use or with variations in blood pressure.

In one study, clamping of the carotid artery reduced rCBF in all patients, except those with collaterals functioning well under hypocapnia [29]. Flow reduction during clamping was homogeneous over the entire cerebral hemisphere. In patients with ischemic foci in the preoperative rCBF studies, the relative flow reductions during clamping in ischemic and nonischemic regions were similar.

STUMP PRESSURE

Stump pressure is another way to measure the adequacy of collateral circulation by clamping the common and external carotid artery on the affected side, and measuring blood pressure in the internal carotid artery distal to the clamping.

Measurement of stump pressure is technically a simple procedure and has been used as an index for safety during carotid endarterectomy. The relationship of stump pressure to systemic blood pressure and rCBF has been evaluated [30–33]. Stump pressure rises proportionately with systemic mean arterial blood pressure, which explains the reasoning for advocating induced hypertension during carotid endarterectomy. Correlation of the effects of induced hypertension on stump pressure and rCBF was good according to Boysen et al. [32]. In reality, however, even though a moderate level of induced hypertension is important during carotid clamping, it does not always prevent neurologic damage in patients with stump pressure below 55 mmHg, which suggests poor collaterals.

The response of stump pressure to $Paco_2$ changes is not uniform. Hypercapnia generally decreased ICA stump pressures even though rCBF measurements during test occlusion show increases in some cases and no changes in others. It may be dangerous in patients with impaired collateral function, in whom a steal may occur with increase in flow only to the unaffected hemisphere. A reduction in stump pressure following carotid artery occlusion under hypercapnia has two etiologic factors: (a) a reduction in pressure in the circle of Willis because of an increase in flow to the opposite hemisphere, and (b) the flow resistance across the collateral channels increasing with increasing flow rates through these vessels.

Hypocapnia when compared to normocapnia gave almost identical ICA stump pressures in patients with poor collaterals, although rCBF values were higher in normocapnic patients. Hypocapnia also did not prevent changes in EEG induced by low rCBF values [34].

In summary, with stump pressures above 70 mmHg during hypocapnia, hypercapnia induces an increased rCBF and a moderate fall in ICA stump pressure. While, during hypocapnia, stump pressure is marginal at 50 mmHg, induction of hypercapnia produces a small increase in rCBF and a proportionate fall in stump pressure. If hypocapnia stump pressure is less than 30 mmHg, rCBF is impaired [35].

Evoked-potential responses and noninvasive carotid studies are the monitoring of the future. They are becoming a more important means of decreasing intraoperative neurologic ischemia. There are still many difficulties to overcome with these monitoring devices. First and foremost is the ability to obtain accurate and easily reproducible signal data for each patient. Second, there are many factors than can affect the somatosensory evoked potential (SEP) average obtained and these factors, such as the use of inhalation anesthetics, are still being identified. A third problem is that, after easily reproducible averages are obtained for each patient, what exactly do small changes in SEP latency and amplitude mean in measurement of reversible and irreversible ischemia? A standardized interpretation of SEP changes is still not available and each center must construct its own protocols and standards of SEP monitoring.

Advances in SEP monitoring, however, are expected to overcome these problems within the next few years with more sensitive instruments and a greater general understanding of the underlying monitoring principles. With increased usage, standards of SEP waveforms can be determined and the importance of changes defined. Dr. B. Grundy in her review article [36] has likened SEP monitoring today to electrocardiogram (ECG) monitoring of a generation ago. Although the equipment is cumbersome and the importance of the small changes in waveform averages is unknown, still in the new few years these difficulties should be resolved. And so, SEP monitoring should become perhaps as a commonplace in the future as ECG monitoring is today.

Most of the methods used to measure possible cerebral ischemia have their limitations. Jugular venous oxygen saturation is not a reliable method of determining regional cerebral ischemia, but will reflect the relationship between total cerebral blood flow and total cerebral oxygen consumption. Stump pressures have been criticized because the values obtained may be influenced by the anesthetic agent and do not change in the same direction as systemic pressures [16]. The EEG has been criticized on the basis of the time lag between vascular occlusion and the appearance of EEG changes indicating major ischemia [20]. The critical cerebral blood flow required to maintain a normal EEG is ~15 ml/ 100 g/min of normal blood flow, which is 30% of normal total blood flow [18]. A flat EEG was obtained with rCBF values of 11 ml/100 g/min during carotid clamping.

Signs of cerebral deterioration during cross-clamping under regional anesthesia include (a) confusion, (b) restlessness, (c) hemiparesis, and (d) seizures.

They indicate clearly that the patient requires shunt placement for adequate perfusion during cross-clamping [21]. Compared to the indirect monitoring techniques employed during general anesthesia, monitoring of motor function and mental state under regional anesthesia give an early and unambiguous indication of when ischemia occurs.

ANATOMY OF CERVICAL PLEXUS

The cervical plexus is formed by the anterior or ventral rami of the upper four cervical nerves. These nerves emerge from the intervertebral foramina of C_1–C_4 and appear in the sulci formed by the anterior and posterior tubercles of the transverse processes. Each nerve receives 1 grey ramus communicantes from the superior cervical ganglion. The nerves exit the sulci and then divide (except for C_1) into ascending and descending branches, which join with adjacent branches to form "loops" that are known as the cervical plexus. The communicating loop from the union of C_2 and C_3, for example, supplies superficial branches to the head and neck while the union of C_3 and C_4 supplies cutaneous innervation to the shoulder and chest [37].

The cervical plexus lies opposite the first four cervical vertebrae, covered by the internal jugular and the sternocleidomastoid, in front of the levator scapulae and scalenus medius. The superificial branches emerge from the posterior border of the sternocleidomastoid and turn cephalad and caudad.

The cervical plexus can further be divided into superficial and deep processes. The superficial branches perforate the cervical fascia and supply skin and sensory information from superficial structures of the neck, shoulder, ear, and posterior scalp. The superficial branches can further be subdivided into ascending and descending processes. Superficial ascending branches include the lesser occipital, the greater auricular, and the anterior cutaneous nerves, all of which supply sensation to the areas of the posterior scalp, neck, and lower mandible. Superficial descending branches from the supraclavicular nerves (medial, intermediate, lateral) supply sensory information from parts of the shoulder and chest to the second rib. The deep cervical plexus branches are divided into medial and lateral processes, which innervate mostly muscle and other deep structures.

CERVICAL PLEXUS BLOCK

The blocks commonly used in anesthesia for carotid artery surgery are deep and superficial cervical plexus blocks [38]. To anesthetize the superficial cervical plexus, the patient is placed in the supine position, with the head extended and rotated away from the side being blocked. A 22-gauge needle is inserted behind the posterior border of the sternocleidomastoid at its midpoint, where the external jugular vein crosses over the muscle. After aspiration, xylocaine 1.5% or similar anesthetic solution may be injected, 2 cc per segment to be blocked (usually 6–8 cc). Onset of action may begin almost immediately and is usually complete within 15 minutes.

For anesthetizing the deep cervical plexus, the patient is placed in the same position again with the head extended and turned away from the side being blocked. The tip of the mastoid process is located and marked, and Chassaignac's tubercle, the anterior tubercle on the transverse process of C_6, is also marked. A line drawn between these two points gives the approximate plane of where the cervical transverse processes are located. The transverse process of C_2 is located by palpating 1.5 cm below the tip of the mastoid process along the previous line drawn and marked. Similarly, the transverse processes of C_3 and C_4 are also palpated and marked along this line, each 1.5 cm apart, below C_2. Skin wheals are raised at these points and $1\frac{1}{2}$-inch 22-gauge needles are inserted perpendicularly and advanced slightly caudad until they rest on the transverse processes. Paresthesias may or may not be elicited. While holding the needle against the transverse process, and after aspiration for blood or cerebospinal fluid, 2 cc of 0.5% Marcaine or similar local anesthetic solution can be injected at each transverse process.

Since the interscalene space freely communicates from C_1 to C_4, another technique is to inject 8–9 cc of 0.5% Marcaine at only one transverse process, with digital compression below C_4 to prevent caudal spread of anesthetic solution to the brachial plexus [39, 40].

After incision, many patients can feel discomfort upon manipulation of the carotid sheath, whose sensory innervation is not always blocked by deep or superficial cervical block. This discomfort can be relieved by infiltrating 2–3 cc of a local anesthetic solution into the carotid sheath prior to any further manipulation.

COMPLICATIONS OF CERVICAL PLEXUS BLOCK

Complications of cervical plexus blocks are related to the vascularity and anatomy of the paravertebral space. Because of the close proximity of the vertebral arteries, intraarterial injection with the onset of convulsions is a significant complication. Intravenous injection and anesthetic uptake may lead to systemic local anesthetic toxicity with hemodynamic instability and central nervous dysfunction, with unconsciousness and convulsions. The local anesthetic can be inadvertently injected into the epidural or subarachnoid space leading to the development of a total spinal block with respiratory and hemodynamic instability. Other complications of cervical plexus block include hematoma formation, cervical sympathetic nerve block, vagal nerve block, facial nerve palsies, recurrent laryngeal nerve paralysis with hoarseness and, when performed bilaterally, bilateral phrenic nerve paralysis [38]. The treatment is symptomatic and those side effects are very transient. Bilateral phrenic nerve paralysis and complete spinal anesthesia require mechanical ventilation.

COMMON MANAGEMENT OF THE PATIENT
UNDER REGIONAL ANESTHESIA

1. Use of intraarterial blood pressure monitoring.
2. Use of modified V_5 ECG lead.
3. Careful head positioning with the head turned away from the operation site and secured with adhesive tape.
4. O_2 via nasal cannula.
5. Careful aspiration prior to injection of the local anesthetic.
6. The effect of 3-min carotid occlusion can be used as an indication for or against the use of a shunt. By using a hand-held "squeaker" by the patient on the opposite side of the site of surgery during cross-clamping, if the patient can still squeeze the toy, his motor function is still intact [41].
7. Avoid deep sedation during carotid cross-clamping.
8. Maintain blood pressure with 10% of preoperative values.

What are the goals of anesthesia for carotid endarterectomy? It should provide analgesia to the patient, thereby facilitating surgery and reducing perioperative morbidity. Emboli and not low perfusion pressure appear to cause most permanent perioperative nervous system dysfunction following carotid endarterectomy. Technical problems account for 40% of cases of intraoperative stroke and embolic phenomena account for another 20%. What we are dealing with, with our anesthetic technique, is about 40% of the complications. Therefore, the anesthetic agent is not the principal factor influencing the outcome of the patients after endarterectomy.

The major cause of mortality and morbidity following carotid endarterectomy is myocardial infarction, with a reported incidence ranging from 0 to 20%. Prough et al. [42] have recently reported a series of 185 carotid endarterectomies performed in 153 patients under regional anesthesia without the development of a perioperative myocardial infarction, although no serial CPK MB studies were routinely ordered. This is far less than what was reported by Tarhan et al. after general anesthesia [43].

Myocardial infarction can occur if the patient becomes hypertensive and has significant heart disease. A strong correlation between the incidence of myocardial infarction and preexisting heart disease, particularly coronary artery disease, has been documented in patients undergoing carotid artery endarterectomy [42, 44–46]. The incidence of myocardial infarction in one series of patients undergoing carotid endarterectomy under regional anesthesia was 0.5% for patients without heart disease, and 4.9% for patients with preexisting heart disease. There were no cardiac deaths as a result of myocardial infarction among operations on patients without heart disease. The use of intraoperative vasopressors during carotid clamping is tolerated well by patients without heart disease, but such drugs increase the incidence of myocardial infarction from 2% to 8.1% among those patients with a history of previous myocardial infarction, congestive heart failure, arrhythmias, angina, or other cardiac disease [46]. Adequate blood pressure should be maintained within 10% of the preoperative range to prevent myocardial infarction. Prompt pharmacologic intervention was the rule for hypertensive as well as hypotensive episodes. Phenylephrine [47] and metaraminol [46] have been used to treat hypotension. Since phenylephrine is a pure alpha-agonist, it produces a reflex bradycardia that may help in maintaining myocardial oxygen demand within acceptable limits. Agents possessing both alpha- and beta-adrenergic agonist effects could more easily produce an imbalance of myocardial oxygen demand and supply in patients who are at risk because of coronary artery disease. The increased incidence of perioperative myocardial infarction reported in patients with heart disease in whom metaraminol was used to maintain blood pressure during carotid artery surgery clamping might reflect this phenomenon [46].

Neurologic deficits following carotid endarterectomy have been reported [47]. It was found that there was a positive correlation between the development of hypertension postoperatively and neurologic deficit. Neurologic deficits were seen in 20% of patients who became hypertensive, compared to 6% in those whose remained normotensive. Patients who had poor blood pressure control preoperatively were more likely to develop hypertension postoperatively than were patients whose blood pressure was well controlled or who were normotensive. Permanent neurologic sequelae occurred far more frequently in patients demonstrated to have bilateral carotid artery disease than in those with unilateral disease.

COMPLICATIONS

Anesthetic complications of significance in this context include hypotension, reflex bradycardia during carotid manipulation, and cardiac arrhythmias. All of these factors may reduce cerebral blood flow. In these patients, because of their age and associated cardiac and respiratory disease, low PaO_2 values are frequently seen preoperatively.

Neurologic damage is probably the most serious complication of this procedure and is related to reduced cerebral blood flow during anesthesia and operation. It may be anything from prolonged unconsciousness due to a transient fall in rCBF, to frank cerebral infarction resulting in stroke.

Postoperative problems unrelated to anesthesia include (2) instability of blood pressure (b) loss of carotid body function, and rarely (c) respiratory insufficiency.

Instability of blood pressure may first appear in the immediate postcarotid occlusion period in the recovery room and occasionally after 24 h. Hypotension or hypertension is reported to occur in about 40% of patients undergoing carotid endarterectomy. In our experience, the incidence is less than 25%. The usual postoperative causes of hypotension such as hypovolemia, acidosis, and cardiac arrhythmias may not account for such hypotension.

The role of carotid sinus reflex as the principal factor in producing blood pressure instability has been reported [35, 48, 49]. Baroreceptor reflex responses to Valsalva's maneuver are reduced in patients with bilateral carotid endarterectomy [49, 50].

Prolonged induced hypertension may reset the baroreceptors so that they respond only to higher blood pressures. Their sensitivity is also reduced following carotid endarterectomy.

Stroke may result from marked hypotension or hypertension in the postoperative period. We routinely treat significant decreases in blood pressure aggressively by infusion of albumin, position changes, or a neosynephrine infusion, and hypertension with vasodilators (sodium nitroprusside, nitroglycerin, or trimethaphan). The goal is to maintain the blood pressure within 10%–15% of the highest preoperative values. Close monitoring is essential to prevent a precipitous fall in blood pressure.

There is a significant loss of carotid body function in cases of bilateral carotid endarterectomy [50]. Normal ventilatory and circulatory responses to hypoxia were reported to be absent in these cases. Increases in Pa_{CO_2}, of 6 mmHg, did not produce any increase in ventilation. The loss of carotid body function many times is not permanent, and it is usually due to transient disturbances of their blood supply intraoperatively.

One of the most fearful complications of carotid endarterectomy is the loss of cardiorespiratory responses to hypoxia. This loss is more dangerous in the chronic obstructive pulmonary disease patient whose ventilation depends on the hypoxic drive. Hypoxia in these patients may produce circulatory collapse instead of the usual hyperventilation and hypervention. This is one reason behind postoperative oxygen therapy for 24 h following carotid endarterectomy.

Respiratory insufficiency in these patients is extremely rare. It is usually due to compression of the upper airway by an expanding hematoma. Unilateral vocal cord paralysis does not lead to respiratory insufficiency unless laryngeal edema occurs.

ADVANTAGES OF REGIONAL ANESTHESIA
FOR CAROTID ENDARTERECTOMY

How good is regional anesthesia for carotid endarterectomy?

Regional anesthesia allows moment-to-moment assessment of neurologic function and avoids the hazards of routine shunting [51–55]. While the evidence is not clear cut, some data support the contention that regional anesthesia offers advantages in possibly lessening the incidence of myocardial infarction, as noted in a recent study at the Bowman Gray School of Medicine [42].

There is a definite correlation between postoperative hypertension and neurologic deficits. During carotid artery occlusion, the blood pressure showed a tendency to rise. This probably was due to the baroreceptor reflexes, which remain intact during local anesthesia in contrast to general anesthetics, which reduce the blood pressure by vasodilatation and myocardial depression. A rise in blood pressure apparently increases the collateral blood flow to the brain and this effect is regarded beneficial [56]. (We don't think regional anesthesia per se will produce a decrease in blood pressure but our general observation confirms that the incidence of hypertension was less following regional anesthesia than general anesthesia in the postoperative period.) The main advantage in using a regional anesthetic is that fewer patients develop postoperative hypertension.

The real advantage of regional anesthesia is that patient consciousness and mental status are the only really foolproof methods to assess adequate cerebral blood flow and oxygenation. The methods for intraoperative assessment of the adequacy of cerebral blood flow are far from reliable, and routine use of shunting under general anesthesia is associated with major complications. Stump pressures show a poor correlation to cerebral blood flow, and both false negatives and positives occur. The EEG may not identify small focal areas of ischemia, and the depth of anesthesia and $Paco_2$ must be held constant to interpret any changes in the EEG. The EEG changes may not occur until severe ischemia is present. Cerebral blood flow measurements are done only in very few centers. General anesthetics can affect the evoked-potential responses. Barbiturates commonly used to protect the brain against ischemia can result in hypotension resulting in myocardial infarction. What better way to assess cerebral blood flow than by talking to an awake patient? This is one of the most compelling reasons to use regional anesthesia—that neurologic function can be assessed immediately postoperatively—as opposed to general anesthesia, because a patient's mental status is always cloudy after general anesthesia.

Use of regional anesthesia also permits significant reductions in operating room time, recovery room time, and postoperative hospital stay. All of these factors help to reduce hospital costs [57].

In summary, advantages of regional anesthesia for carotid endarterectomy are:

1. It is easy to recognize transient neurologic deficits resulting from undetectable emboli dislodged during dissection, which otherwise would likely become permanent subsequent to carotid clamping.
2. There is no race against time as there can be under general anesthesia.
3. It is possible to avoid routine use of shunts and their complications in all patients who tolerate a test occlusion.
4. It provides a conscious and cooperative patient whose neurologic status is the best available monitor of cerebral blood flow in collateral function when carotid blood flow is occluded on the side of operation.
5. It makes a smooth transition from operative to postoperative phase without emergence phenomena.
6. The cardiovascular depression of general anesthesia is avoided.

REFERENCES

1. Cutler RWP: Neurology. In: Rubenstein E, Feldman DD (eds) Scientific American medicine, vol IIX. Scientific American, New York, 1981, pp 1–4.
2. Merrit HH: A textbook of neurology. Lea and Febiger, Philadelphia, 1979, pp 163–205.
3. Kannell WB, Wolf PA, McGee DL, Dawber TR, McNamara P, Castelli WP: Systolic blood pressure, arterial rigidity, and risk of stroke: the Framingham Study. JAMA 245:1225–1229, 1981.
4. Freis ED: The Veterans Administration cooperative study on antihypertensive agents: implications for stroke prevention. Stroke 5:76–77, 1974.
5. McDowell FH: Prevention of subsequent infarctions and transient ischemic attacks. Adv Neurol 25:277–286, 1979.
6. Evans WE, Cooperman M: The significance of asymptomatic unilateral carotid bruits in preoperative patients. Surgery 83:521–522, 1978.
7. Barnes RW, Marszalek PB: Asymptomatic carotid disease in the cardiovascular surgical patient: is prophylactic endarterectomy necessary? Stroke 12:497–500, 1981.
8. Fitch W: Anaesthesia for carotid artery surgery. Br J Anaesth 48:591–796, 1976.
9. Bland JE, Chapman RD, Wylie EJ, et al.: Neurological complications of carotid artery surgery. Ann Surg 171:459, 1979.
10. Galbraith JG: Safeguards in carotid surgery. Surgery 63:1019, 1968.
11. Boysen G: Cerebral hemodynamics in carotid surgery. Acta Neurol Scand 52:1, 1973.
12. Hoedt-Rasmussen K: Regional cerebral blood flow: the intraarterial injection method [thesis]. Acta Neurol Scand [Suppl 27], 1967.
13. Hoedt-Rasmussen K, Sveinsdottie E, Lassen NA: Regional cerebral blood flow in man determined by intraarterial injection of radioactive inert gas. Circ Res 18:237, 1966.
14. Kogure K, Scheinberg P, Fugishima M, et al.: Effects of hypoxia on cerebral autoregulation. Am J Physiol 219:1393, 1970.
15. Sundt TM, Sandok BA, Whisnant JP: Carotid endarterectomy: complications and preoperative assessment of risk. Mayo Clin Proc 50:301–306, 1975.
16. Ackerman RH: Non-invasive carotid evaluation. Stroke 11:675–678, 1980.
17. Larson CP Jr, Ehrenfeld WK, Wade JG, et al.: Jugular venous oxygen saturation as an index of adequacy of cerebral oxygenation. Surgery 62:31, 1967.
18. Sundt TM Jr, Sharbrough FW, Piepgras DG, Kearns TP, Messick JM Jr, O'Fallon WM: Correlation of cerebral blood flow and electroencephalographic changes during carotid endarterectomy: with results of surgery and hemodynamics of cerebral ischemia. Mayo Clin Proc 56:533–543, 1981.
19. Hertzer NR, Beven EG, Greenstreet RL, Humphries AW: Internal carotid artery back pressure, intraoperative shunting, ulcerated atheromata, and the incidence of stroke during carotid endarterectomy. Surgery 83:306–312, 1978.
20. Pearce HJ, Becchetti JJ, Brown JH: Supraorbital photoplethysmographic monitoring during carotid endarterectomy with the use of an internal shunt: an added dimension of safety. Surgery 87:339–342, 1980.
21. Astrup J, Syman L, Branstron NM, et al.: Cortical evoked potential and extracellular K^+ and H^+ at critical levels of brain ischemia. Stroke 8:51–57, 1977.
22. Lyons C, Clark LC, McDowell H, et al.: Cerebral venous oxygen content during carotid thrombinectomy. Ann Surg 160:561, 1964.
23. Waltz AG, Sundt TM, Michenfelder JD: Cerebral blood flow, jugular venous Po_2 and lactate concentration and arterial–venous oxygen content during carotid endarterectomy. Eur Neurol 6:346, 1971/72.
24. Galbraith JG, McDowall HA: Stroke and occlusive cerebrovascular disease: review and surgical results in 265 cases. J Med Assoc State Ala 38:1107, 1969.
25. Meyer JA, Gotoh F, Favale E: Effects of carotid compression on cerebral metabolism and electroencephalogram. Electroencephalogr Clin Neurophysiol 19:362, 1965.
26. Toole JF, Siekert RG, Whisnant JP (eds): Cerebral vascular diseases: transactions of the sixth conference held under the auspices of the American Neurological Association and the American Heart Association Council on Cerebrovascular Disease. Grune and Stratton, New York, 1968.
27. Stern WE: Circulatory adequacy attendant upon carotid artery occlusion. Arch Neurol

21:455, 1969.
28. Thompson JE, Talkington CM: Carotid endarterectomy. Ann Surg 184:1, 1976.
29. Waltz AG: Regional blood flow: responses to changes in arterial pressure and CO_2 tension. In: Toole JF, Siekert RG, Whisnant JP (eds) Cerebral vascular disease. Grune and Stratton, New York, 1968, pp 66–76.
30. Agnoli A, Fieschi C, Prencipe M, et al.: rCBF studies during carotid surgery. In: Russel RWR (ed) Brain and blood flow. Pitman, London, 1971, pp 346–350.
31. Boysen G: Cerebral blood flow measurement as a safeguard during carotid endarterectomy. Stroke 2:1, 1971.
32. Boysen G, Engell HC, Henriksen H: Effect of induced hypertension on internal carotid artery pressure and regional cerebral blood flow during temporary carotid clamping for endarterectomy. Neurology 22:1133, 1972.
33. Fourcade HE, Larson CP Jr, Ehrenfeld WK, et al.: The effects of CO_2 and systemic hypertension on cerebral perfusion during carotid endarterectomy. Anesthesiology 33:383, 1970.
34. Boysen G, Ladegaard-Pedersen HG, et al.: The effects of $Paco_2$ on regional cerebral blood flow and internal carotid artery pressure during carotid clamping. Anesthesiology 35:286, 1971.
35. Larson CP Jr: Anesthesia and the control of cerebral circulation. In: Wylie EJ, Ehrenfeld WK (eds) Extracranial occlusive cerebrovascular disease. WB Saunders, Philadelphia, 1970, pp 152–183.
36. Grundy BL: Monitoring of sensory evoked potentials during neurosurgical operations: methods and applications. Neurosurgery 11:556–573, 1982.
37. Grays Anatomy, Warwick and Williams 35th British Edition. WB Saunders, Philadelphia, 1973.
38. Carron H, Korbonm G, Rowlingson J (eds): Regional anesthesia. Grune and Stratton, New York, 1984.
39. Winnie AP: Interscalene brachial block. Anesth Analg 49:455–456, 1970.
40. Cousins M, Bridenbaug P (eds) Neural blockade. JB Lippincott, 1980.
41. Spielberger L, Turndorf H, Culliford A, Imparato A: Hand held toy squeaker during carotid endarterectomy in the awake patient. Arch Surg 114:103–104, 1979.
42. Prough DS, Scuderi PE, Stullken E, et al.: Myocardial infarction following regional anesthesia for carotid endarterectomy. Can Anaesth Soc J 31:192, 1984.
43. Tarhan S, Moffitt EA, Taylor WF, et al.: Myocardial infarction after general anesthesia. JAMA 220:1451, 1972.
44. Prys-Robert C: Hypertension and anesthesia: fifty years on [editorial]. Anesthesiology 50: 218–214, 1979.
45. Rubio PA, Guinn GA: Myocardial infarction following carotid endarterectomy. Cardiovasc Dis 2:402–404, 1975.
46. Riles TS, Kopelman I, Imparato AM: Myocardial infarction following carotid endarterectomy: a review of 683 operations. Surgery 85:249–252, 1979.
47. Asiddao CB, Donegan JH, Whitsell RC, et al.: Factors associated with perioperative complications during carotid endarterectomy. Anesth Analg 61:631, 1982.
48. Ranson JHC, Imparato AN, Caluss RH, et al.: Factors in the mortality and morbidity associated with surgical treatment of cerebrovascular insufficiency. Circulation [Suppl 1] 39–40: 269–274, 1969.
49. Wade JG, Larson CP Jr, Hickey RF, et al.: Effect of carotid endarterectomy on carotid chemoreceptor and baroreceptor function in man. N Engl J Med 282:823, 1970.
50. Wade HG: Anesthesia for carotid endarterectomy: annual refresher course lecture, no. 208, 1972. American Society of Anesthesiologists Annual Meeting, Boston, 1972.
51. Bosiljevac J, Farha J: Carotid endarterectomy: results using regional anesthesia. Am Surg 46:403–408, 1980.
52. Connolly JE: Carotid endarterectomy in the awake patient. Am J Surg 150:159–164, 1985.
53. Imparato AM, Ramirez A, Riles T, Mintzer R: Cerebral protection in carotid surgery. Arch Surg 117:1073–1078, 1982.
54. Yared I, Martinis A, Mack R: Carotid endarterectomy under local anesthesia: a retrospective study. Am Surg 45:709–71, 1979.
55. Shifrin E, Gertel M, Anner H, Olshwang D, Levy P: Local anesthesia in carotid endarterectomy: an alternative method. Isr J Med Sci 21:511–513, 1985.

56. Fourcade HE, Larson CP, Ehrenfeld WK, Hickey RF, Newton TH: The effects of CO_2 and systemic hypertension on cerebral perfusion pressure during carotid endarterectomy. Anesthesiology 33:383, 1970.
57. Gabelman C, Gann D, Ashworth C, Carney AL: One hundred consecutive carotid reconstructions: local versus general anesthesia. Am J Surg 145:477–471, 1983.

INDEX